Nurse Practitioners in Primary Care

Naomi Chambers

Radcliffe Medical Press

© 1998 Naomi Chambers

Radcliffe Medical Press Ltd
18 Marcham Road, Abingdon, Oxon OX14 1AA, UK

British Library Cataloguing in Publication Data

A catalogue record for this book is available from the British Library.

ISBN 1 85775 298 8

Library of Congress Cataloging-in-Publication Data is available.

Typeset by Acorn Bookwork, Salisbury, Wilts
Printed and bound by Redwood Books, Trowbridge, Wilts

Contents

Preface

The family doctor service, the cornerstone of the NHS, faces unprecedented pressures. As this century draws to a close, there are indications that the public, doctors and nurses are willing to consider breaking the mould that was fixed in the opening years of this century by government legislation. Aimed at a diverse audience, including harassed general practitioners, nurses eager to take on more responsibility and health authority executives facing hard choices about where to invest, as well as students of primary health care, this book examines the potential for nurses providing a first-point-of-contact consultation service as an alternative to going to see the doctor.

In the first part of the book (Chapters 1 and 2) the nature of the pressures encountered by, and the sources of dissatisfaction with, general practitioners are analysed, and the different nurse practitioner models that have been developed across the world are looked at. The rationale for the kind of nurse practitioner proposed as suitable for the UK is presented. This nurse is experienced and offers diagnosis, treatment and advice for minor illness and for other health matters which patients may consider are appropriate for a nurse consultation. These are not triage nurses: they work closely with other colleagues, especially the family doctor, and their work is guided but not bound by protocols. The focus is on a holistic nursing approach to health care, but the medical model of disease management is also used where appropriate.

The second part of the book (Chapters 3, 4 and 5) describes the impact of this nurse on patients, doctors and other nurses, drawing from the results of one study and comparing it with other research in the same field. Three aspects in particular are considered: the consultation experience, the organization of the service, and changes in roles and relationships between doctors and nurses. This section also highlights the problems in primary care which the nurse practitioner concept does not address, and suggests some additional solutions.

In the light of the evidence about the value of nurses as first-point-of-contact primary care providers, the final part of the book (Chapter 6) looks at the nuts and bolts of how the new model can be implemented. The practical steps which policy makers, health authorities, general practitioners and nurses can take to reshape the way in which primary care is delivered using the resource of the nurse practitioner are spelt out.

Naomi Chambers
April 1998

Acknowledgements

This book stems from a PhD thesis undertaken at Manchester University and a primary care development project in Derbyshire. Without the people who took the trouble to complete the patients' surveys, and the health professionals who submitted to the focus group discussions, it would not have been possible. I am also particularly grateful to my supervisor at Manchester University, Rod Sheaff, for his light touch and skilful steer over six years.

Many others have helped and given encouragement including, but not exclusively, the three Derbyshire practices who took part in the project: Martin Cassidy, Hilary Fender, John Habershon, Val Hillier, Keith Houghton, Veronica Marsden, Chris Roberts, Jessie Torrance and Jeffrey Worrall.

Derbyshire Family Practitioner Committee (subsequently Family Health Service Authority and now Southern Derbyshire Health Authority) funded the project and I am grateful for their support.

Finally, Nick Lourie has had to bear the brunt of some of the more difficult moments during the gestation of the thesis and this book, sometimes unwittingly, has helped me to overcome the trickier hurdles.

1 An alternative to seeing the doctor?

Experience as a patient, a mother, a friend and also as a health service manager suggests that there are many occasions when a health problem arises which needs to be queried or talked through with a health professional, but not necessarily with a doctor. This observation is not derived merely from personal and work experiences. It has been found that family doctors consider a third of all consultations to be for trivial, inappropriate or unnecessary reasons (Cartwright and Anderson, 1981). In another study, more than half the doctors questioned felt that the presentation of trivia was a serious problem in general practice (Bowling, 1981). The Cumberlege community nursing review found, from a specially commissioned Marplan survey, that two thirds of the respondents would be prepared to see or talk to a nurse instead of a doctor. Sixty per cent said that they would prefer to see a nurse for certain purposes, and of these, 40% gave as their reason the fact that a nurse was more sympathetic and easier to talk to than a doctor (DHSS, 1986).

It is not surprising that the GP is often the first contact for a wide range of problems, many of which are not strictly medical, given the extent to which physical, emotional and social problems are inextricably related. There is a psychological value for many people in having social contact with the doctor. In view of the cost of their training, however, and the salary differentials between doctors and other health professionals, the question should be asked whether we can continue to afford this kind of open access for consulting over non-medical problems or medical problems which could safely be dealt with by another health professional. Buchan and Richardson (1973) found that 50% of total consultation time had no clinical component and 10% of consultations involved procedures within the competence of a nurse. Half of all illness presented in general practice was described by Fry (1992) as minor, self-limiting and short-lived. In view of the arguments over rationing of health services and the focus on investing in outcomes- and evidence-based health care, should minor, self-limiting and short-lived illness be automatically and routinely dealt with by a professional with gross earnings of £60 000? In the US, where over 15 000 nurse practitioners are employed, it has been suggested that their training costs about one sixth of the amount spent on physicians' training. Although US nurse practitioners spend about 50% more time on each consultation they still represent good value for money (Office of Technology Assessment, 1986).

Despite the potential desirability of direct access to other health professionals, the family doctor system in the UK has changed little since the 1911 National Health Insurance Act, which created the panel, the list of insured patients for whom the doctor was responsible (Honigsbaum, 1979). In particular, the general practitioner's gatekeeping role has remained largely intact. This means that he* is usually the first point of contact in the NHS for people seeking help with some aspect of their health. In addition, patients depend on their GP to refer them to other NHS services. General practice is big business: 99% of the population is registered with a doctor, and 70% of the population consult their doctor at least once a year (Fry, 1992).

Underlying this book is a doubt about the appropriateness of this dually monopolizing role, as first-point-of-contact practitioners in the NHS and as gatekeepers for the rest of the NHS. This role is called into question from a number of health policy angles: the rising costs of the NHS, the increased commitments faced by GPs, the relevance of their training, people's opinions of the family doctor service and the contribution which nurses might often make as a more appropriate point of first contact. The book will develop an alternative model for primary health care, in which the patient could initially choose to consult with either a doctor or a new kind of nurse – a nurse practitioner.

Although there is no agreed definition of the term 'nurse practitioner', there is an emerging view that this nurse is an autonomous professional, with expertise in the diagnosis and management of undifferentiated health problems (Fawcett-Henesy, 1992). There were a number of experiments on the part of nurses in the 1980s to address this issue, the two most notable examples being those of Stilwell (1988) and Burke-Masters (1990, personal communication) (see also Cohen, 1984). The 1990s have seen a growing interest in the potential for nurse practitioners, and the introduction of a number of nurse practitioner diploma courses. This has resulted in a significant increase in the number of nurses calling themselves nurse practitioners and some experimental schemes funded by the Department of Health and Regions. There has not yet been any examination initiated and undertaken from outside nursing and medicine as to the viability and desirability of nurse practitioner-run surgeries. This book aims to fill that gap by pursuing the issue from an organizational rather than a professional perspective, by looking at the results of a study in Derbyshire and by using the mainly nursing work already undertaken in this field as a valuable reference point.

---

*As three out of four general practitioners are men (Statistical Bulletin, Department of Health, 1994), 'he' will be used to mean both male and female general practitioners.

Pressures facing general practitioners

What are the deficiencies of the existing system which a nurse practitioner role may address?

There are many pressures facing general practice at the moment, but five will be highlighted here because of the potential impact which nurse practitioners may bring to bear on them:

- time management problems

- the appropriateness of medical training in the delivery of a modern primary health service

- low morale among GPs

- perceived recruitment problems

- the demands placed on GPs by fundholding and commissioning responsibilities.

The question of time management

In any business, time can be as valuable a resource as money. In the health business, there is an opportunity cost in any decision taken by a family doctor in connection with the allocation of his time. If he decides to carry out the smear tests, rather than another member of the practice team, he has lost the opportunity to spend that time on areas of prevention, diagnosis and treatment which perhaps only a clinician is competent to manage. The work of GPs has been likened to housework: 'it is often ill-defined, can be boundless, and is usually taken for granted' (Richman, 1987). If that is so, effective time management is crucially important and decisions about priorities and suitable areas for delegation should be made explicit.

Concern about time constraints extends to the users of the family doctor service; much of the consumer research in general practice (for example, Cartwright and Anderson, 1981; Age Concern, 1986, Williamson, 1988) suggests that patients worry about wasting the doctor's time, and believe that doctors do not spend enough time with patients. Doctors also worry about not giving enough time to their patients: Cartwright and Anderson reported that doctors were more likely to complain about workload than in their previous study 13 years earlier, despite decreases in list sizes (Cartwright and Anderson, 1981); Bowling found that 62% of doctors surveyed had insufficient time to devote to patients whom they felt needed their attention (Bowling, 1981); and Rice described the time pressures in general practice and the toll which they can take, particularly for those doctors who do try to take time, and who therefore attract patients with emotional and psychological troubles (Rice, 1990). Often, the nub of the problem seems to be the length of the consultation itself. One doctor explains: 'It's a terrible problem. Often by the time I've dealt with the medical problem, we've run out of time so I can't sit and discuss the treatment...' (Rice, 1990). Research shows a positive correlation between the length of the general practitioner consultation and patient satisfaction (Howie *et al.*, 1991).

Given the fact that doctors are chronically short of time and much of what patients come and see doctors about is *clinically* minor and self-limiting, the argument begins to build that nurses could offer an alternative consultation service.

Medical training

The time problems of general practice may be inextricably entangled with the concerns about the competence and confidence of the GP to meet the complex needs of his patients. When doctors indicate that they do not have the time for something, it may be an excuse (as much to themselves as to their patients) for not feeling able or trained to help with the problem presented. 'I worried about their physical progress but had no time, *and no training* [emphasis added], to help me deal with the psychological and emotional aspects of their illness.' This was how Gillian Rice described her feelings about her work with patients as a junior hospital doctor three years after qualifying (Rice, 1990). It might seem unfair to criticize doctors for not being able to cope with every type of situation, given the enormous variety in general practice, until we remember their dual monopoly as the professional of first contact and as the gatekeeper for other NHS professionals and services.

Family doctors also seem particularly concerned about being overwhelmed by trivia, which their training appears not to prepare them for. Cartwright and Anderson discovered that even after 13 years had elapsed, the same proportion of surgery consultations (one third of the total) were considered by the doctors to be for trivial, inappropriate or unnecessary reasons (Cartwright and Anderson, 1981). Trivia, according to the doctors surveyed, included certain specific physical conditions (for example, toothache, colds, sore throats), family and personal problems, and form-filling. In the later study, a larger proportion of doctors (87% as compared with 67%) felt it was inappropriate for patients to seek help with family problems. What doctors do not reveal is where, if anywhere, patients should take these kinds of problems. Bowling discovered that over half the doctors in her study felt that the presentation of trivia was a serious problem in general practice (Bowling, 1981). The amount of trivia was felt by some of the doctors in Bowling's sample to threaten their clinical expertise. It was the doctors with a lesser interest in psychiatry and in the treatment of emotional problems who were most concerned.

A brief examination of undergraduate medical training reveals that there is little time spent on managing the emotional and psychological aspects of illness. And yet, as seen earlier, Buchan and Richardson found that 50% of GP consultation time had no clinical component at all (Buchan and Richardson, 1973). This suggests that skills other than clinical expertise have to be acquired by doctors, and indeed by nurse practitioners, if they are to share first-point-of-contact health care in the future. Despite the recommendation of the General Medical Council (GMC) in 1980 that, on graduation, a medical student should be able to communicate effectively and sensitively with patients and their relatives, a GMC working party seven years later found that the recommendation had not been strong enough to develop the proper teaching of communication skills. Efforts continue to be made to address criticisms that doctors are ineffective communicators. By 1993 the GMC was able to report improvements in teaching in this area, while reiterating the importance of building on these improvements and noting the contribution that other health professionals make in the field of communications (GMC, 1993).

A further problem lies in the location and focus of undergraduate medical training, as lacking the proper perspective of illness in the community. A King's Fund report in 1994 described an initiative to introduce community-based medical education devised by King's College Medical School and noted enormous interest in this project but little action on the part of other medical schools (Seabrook et al., 1994). It would appear that despite a recognition of the problem, alternative visions and innovative projects, undergraduate medical education is still, on the whole, hospital and secondary care focused and therefore poor preparation for addressing the problems which patients bring in primary health care.

According to Rice, the problem lies not only in the curriculum, but in the ethos of the hospital-based medical school, which teaches the ridiculing of ignorance and the inappropriateness of admitting to inexperience (Rice, 1990). The role models for junior doctors are the consultants who have 'survived' the system and who see 'good' doctors as the ones who are tough and resilient, not the ones who get distressed over the enormity of their new responsibilities and their inhumanly long working hours. Worryingly, housemen look to their seniors, not to their patients, for a judgement on their performance. Although the GP vocational training scheme has significantly upgraded training, it should be remembered that two out of the three years on the scheme are spent in the hospital environment, as junior doctors working in the prevailing culture described above.

Proposals for changes to the vocational training scheme for GPs coming from both within and outside the profession (NAHAT, 1994; RCGP, 1994) suggest that the current arrangements are inadequate to meet the clinical and organizational demands which today's GP is facing. The National Association of Health Authorities and Trusts (NAHAT, now the NHS Confederation), for example, argued that vocational training should be increased from three to five years, and that the MRCGP examination, currently optional, should be the normal standard for GP principals. As the vocational training scheme only became mandatory in 1981, and general practice is a career 'for life', many practising GP principals have no specialized training for general practice, let alone five years. It follows that many patients may not be receiving care from appropriately trained doctors.

There is also an issue surrounding the connection between gender and the patient-centredness of general practice consultations. The patient-centred method focuses on understanding the patient's reason for consulting and their expectations for the outcome: it involves entering the patient's world and seeing the illness through their eyes. The method can be measured by taping consultations and then scoring doctors' responses to the patients' contributions to the consultation, and doctors' efforts at encouraging the expression of the patients' thoughts, feelings and expectations. A review of the literature reveals increasing evidence that this approach achieves improved patient satisfaction, better control of symptoms and speedier recovery. The research associated with the review found that women GPs were more patient-centred than men GPs, and women trainers were more patient-centred than other women GPs. The research also found that women practitioners' patient-centredness scores were higher with female patients than with male patients, and the lowest scores were male practitioners with female patients (Law and Britten, 1995). These results pose a problem: women GP trainers are rarer than women principals, who themselves only account for one in four GPs (Department of Health Statistical Bulletin, 1994), but women consistently consult more frequently than men (General Household Survey, 1992). A number of solutions come to mind: better medical training in the patient-centred approach, better incentives for women practitioners and trainers or the development and deployment of non-medical women practitioners in the first-point-of-contact role.

On a broader front, there has been an increasingly vocal movement within medical sociology about the effectiveness of the conventional medical model in the treatment of today's health complaints.

Dubos developed the concept of the 'mirage' of health: that it was a dangerous error to believe that disease and suffering could be wiped out by new therapeutic procedures or higher standards of living because, as the world changed, there was a new burden of diseases created by the failure of humankind to adapt biologically and socially to the changes (Dubos, 1968). This suggests that we may be pursuing unrealistic goals in allowing our primary health care system to be medically led. McKeown asserts that external environment and personal behaviour are more important factors in determining health than the provision of curative medical services, which suggests that our structures and priorities for investment in primary health care are wrong; currently the nurses, with their focus on holistic care and health promotion, support the doctors' work and are paid less (McKeown, 1979).

It has been argued that the current medical model was designed to fit the beliefs and meet the requirements of a century ago, and is overdue for replacement (Inglis, 1981). The focus for medical attention and innovation is on an increasingly narrow range of treatments, with lack of real progress on the common, chronic and terminal diseases, such as backache, arthritis and cancer. Inglis writes: '...a great deal of what the profession does is valuable and essential ... but the net value of orthodox medical treatment is far less than it was 25 years ago, and is declining...'. Illich goes further: 'The medical establishment has become a major threat to health. The disabling impact of professional control over medicine has reached the proportions of an epidemic...' (Illich, 1976).

These views add up to a compelling argument that our current structure, which places doctors as sole first-point-of-contact health carers, is not fulfilling society's health needs. Tudor Hart still sees a central place for doctors, but operating under a new set of principles and beliefs (Tudor Hart, 1988). Within the general practice profession itself Tudor Hart proposes a 'new kind of doctor' who practises six features of a medical professionalism:

- an open style of medicine admitting to patients and to colleagues what is not known and cannot be done

- imaginative not uncritical application of scientific principles

- handling health and disease as being on a continuum, not separate entities

- acceptance that effective care and conservation of health depend on skills of other health professionals as well as doctors

- view of patients as colleagues, not passive consumers of care

- alliance with ordinary people, not establishment.

The 'new doctor' may be what is required, but how far is the medical profession from this ideal?

Meanwhile, what potential is there for a 'new kind of doctor' and a 'new kind of nurse' to work together as a team in partnership with patients to provide primary health care?

Low morale and burnout

The general practitioner in the nineties has a more task-sensitive contract, yet has continuing 24 hour responsibility to a patient list, and a burgeoning network of paramedical, social and lay experts with whom he/she is expected to communicate to provide a network of primary provision: curing, caring, rehabilitating, preventing and health promoting. The past emphasis on the continuing doctor–patient relationship is being displaced by an emphasis on teamwork, teambuilding, consumerism, networking, computer-aided communications, sophisticated purchasing skills and commercial incentives ... is the breadth of skills demanded of the new general practitioner so wide that a crash is inevitable? (Stott, 1994)

As the quote above demonstrates, there is considerable concern about work and role overload in general practice The medical journals now outline and debate regularly the stresses of working as a GP, for example Petchey's work on young GPs' orientations to change (Petchey, 1994), the RCGP's initiative on 'revaluing general practice' (McBride and Metcalfe, 1995), and general practitioner 'burnout' (Kirwan and Armstrong, 1995). Recruitment into general practice is now more difficult than it has been for years, and in many areas it is proving hard to find locums to cover holidays and sickness. One health authority has introduced a sabbatical scheme to address the issue of recruitment and falling morale among GPs, giving partners up to three months away from the practice with full locum cover from a pool of local GP registrars, who have completed their vocational training but are not yet ready to enter into a commitment of full-time career principal (Munro and Gibbs, 1997).

One of the problems for GPs is that successive reforms have brought them into the NHS centre stage as commissioners of services and shapers of policy at local level, while still requiring them to be full-time clinicians.

NHS reforms

The first challenge from the NHS reforms for GPs came with the imposition of the new GP contract in 1990. Pressure was put on doctors through this contract in a number of areas. Levels of remuneration became more dependent on list sizes than before; some practices began to take on more patients than they could reasonably cope with in order to pay back debts incurred when purchasing new surgeries in the 1980s before the property market collapsed. New health promotion payment systems, targets for screening and immunization, and minor surgery payments all meant recruiting new practice nursing staff and running extra clinics. Hours of availability were more closely defined and expected to match patient demand. Doctors were exhorted to examine their clinical practice through medical audit.

The new contract precipitated a change in the culture of practice organization for many practices from the informal, almost family-run business to a larger, more formal and more bureacratic setup. With more staff to manage, it became necessary to have a practice manager, if there was not one in place already. Not being well schooled in professional recruitment processes, practices often promoted their favourite receptionist and then wondered why she (almost invariably a woman) did not live up to their new expectations. Complex practice finances, medical audit, screening and immunization targets, repeat prescribing and annual report requirements all contributed to a pressure for computerization; this again required staff with new kinds of skills or comprehensive retraining of existing staff, and not all partners were computer-literate either. Family health service authorities (FHSAs) and their successor health authorities introduced practice-based staff and training budgets and began to require development plans for practices before deciding whether to invest in more staff from their cash-limited general medical services (GMS) budget; a business planning culture was being introduced from above. Some practices were already running services and systems in a way required by the new contract before it was in place, but for others, small and large, the changes have been stressful and doctors have felt largely unsupported.

The new contract had not had time to 'bed down' before the next wave of reforms impacted on general practice: the creation of the internal market in April 1991, with purchasers and providers, contracts and service specifications, extra contractual referrals and fundholding. Some practices were keen to enter fundholding, having the management capability and the eagerness to influence changes in the hospital sector for the benefit of their patients. Others entered for fear of being left behind or because they were attracted by the management allowance; this financial incentive later gained the nickname of the 'golden handcuff', because those not really coping with fundholding could not withdraw as they had become dependent on the management allowance. Fundholding meant managing budgets, manipulating patient-throughput data, negotiating contract terms, monitoring quality and, increasingly, working with other practices to get a better 'deal' for patients.

For those who did not sign up to fundholding there was the option to join commissioning groups or local purchasing groups of one kind or another; the technicalities of contracting were left to the health authorities but it was up to the groups to decide what range of services they wanted. This again involves 'above-practice' working and time away from patients or practice administration to attend meetings and write papers.

The internal market was followed through with the concept of the 'primary care-led NHS', in 1994. There were at least two interpretations of this notion. The first inferred that, judging from the success of practice-based minor surgery sessions and the purchase through fundholding of more locally provided or practice-based specialist services (for example, consultant outpatient clinics and physiotherapy), as much care should be provided at the primary level as possible. Some commentators have cast doubt on the efficacy and cost effectiveness of providing some of these services within primary care (for example, Robinson *et al.*, 1997). A reaction from part of the profession has been the 'core and non-core work' debate, suggesting a work-to-rule, which could lead us back to some of the issues raised in the family doctor service in the troubled 1960s. The second interpretation of the concept suggests that all GPs, whether fundholding or not, have a part to play in deciding what kind and range of hospital services should be developed for their patients. The form of that decision making was left to local discretion, until the White Paper *The New NHS* in 1997, which described four different levels of maturity for local primary care groups, which will subsume fundholding in April 1999 (NHS Executive, 1997).

A further initiative to hit GPs was the 1996 White Paper *Choice and Opportunity*, which was followed by the Primary Care Act of 1997, enabling practices and health authorities, if they wished, to throw away the Red Book which regulates the national family health service practitioner contract, and to start with a clean sheet of paper in deciding what primary care services should be provided. Not surprisingly, the flow of submission of pilots to pursue this course has been sluggish. There is concern about a management vacuum in primary care, but surely it must also be a case of a surfeit of new intiatives, with GPs crying out 'Enough . . . no more!'.

Sources of patient dissatisfaction

Hannu Vuori, from the viewpoint of the World Health Organization (WHO), has argued that patients are the ultimate authorities on the criteria of good care (Vuori, 1987). Vuori identifies three areas of care with measurable characteristics that may influence patient satisfaction:

- the science of medicine (technical knowledge and skills)
- the art of care (interpersonal and communication skills)
- the amenities of care (setting, conditions and access).

He also argues that patient satisfaction is an indicator, an attribute and a prerequisite for quality care because care can clearly *not* be of high quality in the absence of patient satisfaction. Patients do appreciate the importance of the technical quality of the care they receive and satisfied patients are more likely to cooperate with their practitioners' proposed treatment plan and to return to seek care again when necessary. Dissatisfaction is a separate entity, but it is important to identify what factors cause dissatisfaction. Vuori summarizes the relative importance of the patients' view: 'The difference between the role of the physician and that of the patient in quality assurance resembles that between the hen and the pig in the preparation of bacon and eggs: the hen is involved but the pig is committed.'

This may be an inelegant way of summarizing the argument, but Vuori's metaphor focuses clearly on the relative importance of the patients' perspective. In Watkins' review of the measurement of quality in general practitioner care he concludes that agreement about what constitutes the criteria for good primary medical care may be far off, but reminds us of one of the earliest examples of quality control in medicine, the Hippocratic oath, which focuses on the importance of a satisfactory relationship between the doctor and his patient (Watkins, 1981).

On the question of practice organization, patients feel strongly about waiting times for an appointment and waiting times at the surgery (Williamson, 1988; Jacoby, 1989; Lewis and Williamson, 1995). A national patients survey of general practice in 1989 found that 17% of patients felt that they had to wait an unreasonable length of time for a non-urgent appointment. A study by the Consumers' Association in 1995 found that patients' top priorities for improvement to the family doctor service were shorter waits for appointments and at the surgery (*Which?*, 1995). The launch of the Patient's Charter initiative has raised expectations generally for NHS patients around issues of access and waiting times. Because of GPs' independent contractor status, and the fact that patient charters were not within the terms and conditions of the national contract, the extension of the charter into primary care was encouraged, but has remained voluntary. As far as patients are concerned, however, they tend not to make distinctions between the various parts of the health service, and there is anecdotal evidence that the ethos of the Patient's Charter intiative has raised patient expectations of family practitioner services. The emerging picture, therefore, is a national consumerist drive, which is encouraging the enforcement of patients' rights and standards of service. This is matched by an uneven response to obtaining a perspective of users' views and no coordinated strategy for dealing with the issues that are uncovered by the examination of the users' perspective.

Above all, patients want doctors with good listening and counselling skills. This is not new. In a report for the Research Institute for Consumer

Affairs in 1963, Hutchinson found that the elements of awe and wonder in the doctor–patient relationship were being transferred from the family doctor with his black bag to the hospital specialist with his miracle drugs and his mastery of intricate skills. But this survey showed that people still wanted mental and spiritual support from their family doctors. Patients had a high opinion of their doctor's medical skills, but were less favourable in their views of his friendliness, understanding and willingness to take time (Hutchinson, 1963). Ten years later, the Patients' Association found that patients tended to judge the quality of the clinical attention they were getting by outward signs which seem irrelevant to the better informed. The same report also found that the GP receptionist was sometimes seen as a filter to ward off patients who did not really need to see the doctor. This suggests a kind of triage well before the term came into use. If *de facto* triage already exists, perhaps it would be preferable if it were to be carried out by a nurse rather than a clinically untrained receptionist; however, the report also suggests that nursing or anything other than medical triage is not likely to be acceptable to patients (Patients' Association, 1973).

In a policy paper written in 1986 about GPs and the needs of older people, Age Concern points out that 40% of the average GP's patient consultations are with elderly people, and suggests that provided patients also have access to a GP as and when necessary, they should have the opportunity of direct access to other staff for advice (Age Concern, 1986). Another client group who are heavy users of the GP service are mothers of small children. In a survey conducted by Brighton Community Health Council (CHC), it was found that 27% of mothers reported intervention on the part of receptionists to discuss the necessity for surgery appointments, 27% were not satisfied with the amount of information they were given regarding treatment and there was a strong feeling of being rushed and that doctors did not listen (Williamson, 1988). Sixty nine per cent of the mothers were willing to be referred directly to the nurse under certain circumstances, and of those, 40% mentioned minor complaints as an appropriate example.

In response to the publication of the Primary Health Care Green Paper in 1986, which advocated the payment of a 'good' practice allowance, *Which?* carried out a survey to find out what patients and doctors thought were important characteristics of a good practice. It was taken for granted that the single most important outcome was that the medical problem was skilfully and properly dealt with. Patients put the doctor's attitude at the top of the list, followed by the explanation of the problem and then the explanation of the treatment. Doctors, on the other hand, thought that the training of receptionists and the organization of the medical records were more important than the doctor's attitude. On the question of practice services that patients considered most important, a practice nurse was the highest priority, followed by the provision of physical check-ups. Doctors considered that the provision of clinics and screening facilities were more important (*Which?*, 1987).

In the doctor–patient relationship, patients most value the doctor's willingness to listen, take time, explain things fully and be sympathetic (Cartwright, 1981; Jacoby, 1989; Calnan and Williams, 1991; *Which?*, 1995). In terms of patient satisfaction, the success of consultations seems to be dependent as much on the doctor's attitude as on the clinical outcome (Williamson, 1988; Rice, 1990). In Baker's work to develop a standardized questionnaire to assess patients' satisfaction with consultations in general practice, he identified three principal factors affecting satisfaction with the consultation: professional care, which included examination and provision of information, depth of the relationship, which included the doctor's intimate knowledge of the patient, and perceived time, concerning the patients' perceptions of the length of consultations when related to their own requirements (Baker, 1990). In a subsequent study to develop a standard multidimensional patient satisfaction questionnaire for general practice, Grogan and colleagues, building on Baker's work, found that patients' satisfaction with the practice was far more significantly affected by their doctor than by anything else: the 'doctors' subscale explained 39.4% of variability in satisfaction scores, in contrast with access (which includes the role of the receptionist) which scored 6%, nurses 4.7%, appointments 3.9% and facilities 3.6% (Grogan *et al.*, 1995). But, using principal components analysis, Grogan also found (unlike Baker) that patients did not discriminate between different aspects of the consultation in terms of satisfaction, and that getting appointments constituted a separate factor from other related areas such as 'access' (Grogan, 1995).

There are some differences in the findings from patient surveys over recent years, but the literature consistently produces two recurring major themes: the availability of appointments and the style and content of the GP consultation. The main complaints are lack of time with the doctor, a lack of information and explanation, and the erection of barriers, from receptionists to appointment systems, preventing people from seeing the doctor. In addition to the Patient's Charter initiative, trends can be detected which suggest that patients are gradually less accepting of the situation. The second Cartwright study found that patients were likely to be more critical than 13 years earlier (Cartwright, 1981). Patients are still generally satisfied with services provided by their GP, but the picture is one of heightened expectations and growing dissatisfaction.

To remedy this deteriorating situation in general practice, would patients find the nurse practitioner acceptable as an alternative first point of contact? It is hard to be sure about this, as patients tend to prefer what is, rather than a possible future option which they have not experienced. There are clues in the literature, however.

An earlier survey, which aimed to map the accessibility of primary health care services, also found an acceptance of the idea of seeing the nurse instead of the doctor. Seventy one per cent of people who had intended to see the doctor, but who saw a nurse or health visitor instead, said they did not mind who they saw, 20% would have preferred to see the nurse anyway and 9% would have preferred to see the doctor (Ritchie *et al.*, 1981).

The Brighton CHC survey of mothers with pre-school children (Williamson, 1988) found that over two thirds of their sample were willing to be seen initially by the nurse under certain circumstances, especially for minor complaints. Actual experience of consulting the nurse was associated with a higher level of acceptance of her extended role, which mirrors the results in the US. Williamson provides the following interpretation of the Brighton survey:

> The findings suggest that there may be room for considerable expansion of the role of the nurse, but that some education of patients may be necessary to convince the sizeable reluctant minority that it is an appropriate procedure. It is interesting to note that 80% of those who had already consulted the practice nurse and who were satisfied with the treatment they received from her, were content to be referred direct. This suggests that direct experience can be quite effective in inducing acceptance. (Williamson, 1988)

The research literature suggests therefore that patients would accept the idea of the nurse practitioner. It is not clear how far they would *welcome* a new model for providing health care in the practice setting. The different possible models are described in the following chapter, with an analysis of which is likely to be most acceptable to the professions and to government.

2 Nurse practitioners for the UK

Alternative nurse practitioner models

The term 'nurse practitioner' was coined in the US, in the early 1960s, when a shortage of primary doctors in Colorado forced the introduction of the new health care worker, initially in the area of paediatrics (Bliss and Cohen, 1977). At the beginning of the 1980s there were 18 000–20 000 nurse practitioners across the US, specializing in a number of areas, including geriatrics, gynaecology and midwifery. By the mid-1980s their numbers had dipped slightly to 15 400 (Office of Technology Assessment, 1986). A national study in the late 1970s showed that 90% of nurse practitioners were white women and were predominantly found in inner city and rural locations, suggesting that they were probably delivering primary care services to underserved populations as a substitute for primary doctors. Wysocki reported nurse practitioners who wanted to work in rural areas received a major filip when Congress enacted the Rural Health Clinic Act in 1977 (Wysocki, 1990). The Act provided for Medicare and Medicaid reimbursement to nurse practitioners, certified nurse midwives and physician's assistants working in rural, medically underserved areas. Fifty per cent of the services in rural health clinics could be provided by these professionals and the clinics could be nurse practitioner owned. However, the Act has met with less success than originally hoped, with only 455 clinics participating by 1988 rather than the several thousand that had originally been projected by that year. The main barriers to further progress are seen as restrictive state practices and reimbursement arrangements and a lack of concrete evidence about the net costs of nurse practitioner services.

Nurse practitioners in the US have an extended nursing function *and* a role in meeting the diagnostic and treatment needs of patients. Their work includes physical examinations, counselling, teaching, referrals, dealing with chronic disease and minor illnesses, and some prescribing. The work which they initially took on has been described thus: 'The first patients that nurse practitioners were allowed to add to their caseloads were the undesirables – the old, the poor, the alcoholic, the mentally ill, the noncompliant. Therefore, nurses quickly found themselves caring for the sickest patients, not the healthiest' (Diers and Molde, 1983). Not surprisingly, in view of this work profile, their greatest fear in the early days was of killing a patient, and Diers and Molde report that the nurses were obsessed with knowing everything about anything which could go wrong with the body. As their confidence grew, the emphasis switched to holistic care, incorporating lessons learnt from their nurse training, although careful diagnosis and treatment management are still considered important. Their role has been considered as complementary to that of the physician:

> The nurse practitioner and the physician form the dyad of principal health and illness care providers in primary care... As he [the doctor] is occupied with illness care, the nurse practitioner deals with the patients' health maintenance, health education, attainment of higher levels of health, and the achievement of a dignified, peaceful death. Manifestly, there is an overlap of functions between the physician and the nurse practitioner in the area of physical assessment and in the management of simple and common illnesses. (Mauksch, 1978)

Although the role of the nurse practitioner has been relatively well accepted in the management of certain common episodic and chronic health problems of individuals and families in the US, following specialty-based training, Fenton and others have argued that nurse practitioners have not generally taken leadership roles in the community in the provision of the full range of primary health care, because of a lack of appropriate broader-based training (Fenton et al., 1991). Conversely, community health nurses are trained to assess, plan and perform health care and promotion activities with populations and aggregates in the community, but are not trained to manage common health problems, and refer patients to physicians for simple health matters. They have proposed a solution which involves a masters-level nurse practitioner training programme, encompassing the skills of both these types of nurses and allowing students to choose a clinical speciality area, while providing all students with a foundation in primary health care for all age groups, and family and community health concepts. This approach appears remarkably close to the community nurse training proposed by the UKCC, in which all nurses gain a community nursing qualification and also specialize (for example in health visiting or district nursing).

There have been a number of arguments marshalled in favour of the US nurse practitioner role. On the economic side, Lancaster and Lancaster argue that: '... there is little logic in a health care system that uses the most skilled workers as the gatekeepers to the system. Why have we not developed a more cost-effective system for the health care division of labour?' (Lancaster and Lancaster, 1993:3). Mundinger further argues that nurse practitioners are also cheaper because they select less costly treatment options (Mundinger, 1994). On manpower planning, Lancaster and Lancaster argue that it is becoming clear that the current numbers and mix of health professionals cannot meet the current, much less the future, expanded need for primary health care services. Both Lancaster and Lancaster and Mundinger suggest that in the future doctors should be trained for speciality rather than primary care, on the basis that there is a growing gap between the specialist and primary care physicians and a growing overlap in practice between the primary care physicians and nurse practitioners. Others argue that the medical generalist cannot be allowed to disappear (Petersdorf, 1992; Colwill, 1992). But there is also an emerging consensus that the way forward is not nurse practitioners working autonomously and in conflict about 'turf' with physicians, but a collaborative teamwork approach in which nurse practitioners diagnose and manage uncomplicated illnesses, with doctors still primary in complex and critical cases. However, it is not clear whether these physicians are specialists, subspecialists or the primary care physicians (Lancaster and Lancaster, 1993; Kassirer, 1994; Mundinger, 1994).

Research has shown that nurse practitioners in the US can provide high quality primary health care. There were numerous studies conducted in the 1970s and 1980s examining this issue as the nurse practitioner movement developed. Indeed, Lancaster and Lancaster argue that there have been more studies evaluating nurse practitioners' quality of care than that provided by their physician colleagues, that none of the studies detail problems in the performance of nurse practitioners, regardless of their level of preparation, and that many studies demonstrate not only competence but also a high level of patient satisfaction with their services (Lancaster and Lancaster, 1993). There is also evidence in the US of decreased morbidity, lower hospitalization rates and higher patient compliance among the clients cared for by nurse practitioners (reported by the Office of Health Technology Assessment, 1986). The kinds of outcome measures used to examine the nurses' impact included the rate of patient return to employment, reduction in the number and severity of symptoms, and reduction in pain and discomfort. The Office of Health Technology Assessment's report indicates also that the nurses prescribe less frequently than physicians and use well-known and simple drugs. They are particularly good at assisting patients with hypertension and obesity. They 'appear to have better communication, counselling and interviewing skills than physicians have'. Physicians do, however, provide better care in managing problems which require technical solutions.

There is also a high degree of acceptance of and satisfaction with nurse practitioner performance on the part of their employers, doctors, and the patients themselves. Physicians who work with nurse practitioners express more satisfaction with their performance and more willingness to delegate higher level tasks than do physicians whose contact is indirect or non-existent. Patients are particularly satisfied with the care received from nurse practitioners in terms of the personal interest exhibited by the nurse, reduction in the professional mystique of health care delivery and the amount of information conveyed. They were also appreciative of the lower costs. The only area where there was some dissatisfaction reported was with nurse practitioners who did not consult with physicians about diagnostic and treatment decisions.

On the face of it, the development of the nurse practitioner movement in the US appears to be a success story, providing the opportunity for more, better and cheaper primary care in collaboration with physicians. The jury is still out, however. It has been argued that the research to date in this area is incomplete, with a lack of focus on either randomization or cost effectiveness (Brown and Grimes, 1995). The attitude of some physicians remains suspicious. Kassirer has argued against the development of nurse practitioners as fully independent because of the lack of evidence that this mode of practice is efficacious and safe (Kassirer, 1994). Although arguing cautiously for a model of collaborative practice, he points out that nurse practitioners may not be cheaper or more effective: how can they be when they have had shorter training? Other physicians are more enthusiastic about sharing in primary care provision (Shurin, 1993). Even those who approve of the concept express only limited interest in employing nurse practitioners (Office of Health Techology Assessment, 1986). In addition, legal restrictions (especially on prescribing – the situation varies from state to state), the costs of malpractice insurance, and the limitations on coverage and payment for interpersonal and preventive care are all cited as hindrances to further development (Devereaux, 1991; Lancaster and Lancaster, 1993).

The situation in Canada is similar, although there was never a shortage of primary care physicians. The nurse practitioner role developed in the early 1970s, and has always been seen as complementary to, rather than substituting, for the doctor (Jones, 1984), except in very isolated communities. The expanded role includes history taking, physical examination and management of certain aspects of treatment. A recent judgement in Alberta has revealed a double standard about what is an acceptable role for the Canadian nurse practitioner. In a story which is reminiscent of Barbara Burke-Masters' experience in the UK in the 1980s (see below), a nurse practitioner was barred from seeing patients independently and carrying out physical examinations in a city clinic, although she had successfully claimed for years when doing the same work in remote aboriginal settlements (O'Meara, 1994).

Research in Canada has shown that in terms of quality of care and patient acceptability, the nurse practitioners have scored well (Jones, 1984; Spitzer, 1984). The most famous of the studies is the Burlington randomized trial of 1974. Two nurses underwent short training to increase their decision-making and clinical judgement skills. These skills were compared with two family physicians in a suburban practice. Families were randomly allocated to the two nurse practitioners and the two physicians, and then information was obtained from patients, via a questionnaire, about change in health status, use of and satisfaction with services. Adequacy of care management and clinical judgement were inferred from a retrospective assessment of the management of ten common conditions and an evaluation of the manner in which 13 common drugs were prescribed. Results showed an equivalent performance in the management of patients and in patient satisfaction (Spitzer *et al.*, 1974).

A subsequent review of 21 studies directly comparing nurse practitioners and physicians found equivalent performance in all (Sox, 1979). One study examined the quality of medical care provided in five family practices *before* and *after* attachment by 'family practice nurses' and found from an examination of tracer conditions and use of drugs – a similar evaluation method to that used in the Burlington trial – that the standards of patient care had been maintained (Chambers *et al.*, 1978). The Burlington study has, however, been criticized as inadequate for methodological reasons (Kassirer, 1994), and Openshaw questioned the assumption that there is an overall relationship between the management of the presenting problem and the outcome for the patient (Openshaw, 1984). In her view, too little is known about the clinical efficacy of treatments, which is required before the overall adequacy of care by different professionals can be measured.

The barriers to the development of nurse practitioners have seemed more insuperable in Canada than in the US – as well as problems of reimbursement to third parties in the Canadian health care system, and reluctance on the part of the physicians, there is also a surplus of physicians, a continuing concentration of resources on disease-oriented, hospital-centred health care, and a paucity of research addressing health-related outcomes of care (Jones, 1984). During the 1980s there was a curtailment in the educational programmes for nurse practitioners, but this situation appears to be reversing with reports of new programmes now being set up (O'Meara, 1994).

Writing about both the US and Canada in 1984, Spitzer is pessimistic about the long-term viability of the concept: 'Internecine fighting about turf, status, role, and the type of degrees required for safety and effectiveness must be settled.' The Health Technology Assessment Report for the US two years later is more sanguine, without, however, offering any vision of the future. There appears to be a disparity in North America between the considerable body of evidence that nurse practitioner care can be cheaper and as equally effective as physician care, and the actual development and deployment of nurse practitioners.

There has been no nurse practitioner movement in the UK to compare with the movement in North America and elsewhere. Instead there are a small number of interested individuals who have experimented with different models, and a growing acknowledgement from the professions, the academic institutions and government review bodies that nurse practitioners may have a significant part to play.

Barbara Stilwell is perhaps the most well-known UK nurse practitioner. Her experience as a nurse practitioner working in a separate consulting room but alongside other doctors in an inner city Birmingham practice from 1982 to 1985 is well documented (Stilwell, 1982, 1984, 1988). She took the American model, including examination, diagnosis and treatment, and added a focus on long-term health goals. If a prescription was needed, arrangements were made for one of the GPs to sign it. In fact, only 15% of the consultations resulted in a prescription being issued. Stilwell found that the nurse practitioner acted as an alternative health practitioner for patients. She was a particularly popular choice for the women patients of the practice. Patients tended to choose to see Stilwell for advice and preventive health matters, but a third of all consultations were in connection with the management of chronic ailments. And over one third of consultations were with patients presenting with new problems, ranging from mental disorders to genitourinary complaints.

More recently, Stilwell conducted research into the special skills which nurses have to offer and the usefulness of an expanded role for nurses in general practice. The aim was to inform the curriculum for the RCN diploma course. She identified six key functions of a nurse practitioner (Stilwell, 1991:70–1):

- provision of direct access service for patients

- comprehensive assessment including physical examination

- discrimination between normal and abnormal findings

- organization of appropriate screening programmes

- employment of relevant social and communications skills

- limited prescribing.

Stilwell concludes that the role of a nurse practitioner is defined not merely by transference of tasks, but by an autonomy of practice involving case management and time organization (Stilwell, 1991).

Barbara Burke-Masters also worked as a nurse practitioner, but on her own, providing health care, including prescribing and direct referrals to hospitals, to single homeless men in east London from 1982 to 1988. Burke-Masters was partly inspired by her previous experience as a missionary nurse, working in a rural TB hospital in South Africa where a doctor appeared only every two months. Burke-Masters explained her role in the East End as being clearly a substitute doctor (Cohen, 1984). Burke-Masters ran into considerable opposition from the medical profession and from the Pharmaceutical Society. The RCN eventually, but without enthusiasm, granted indemnity insurance to her for all aspects of her work. The voluntary organizations who had hired her in the first place finally withdrew their support, because her model did not allow for teamworking (Burke-Masters, 1990, personal communication).

In 1992, SE Thames Regional Health Authority and the Department of Health funded a project evaluating nurse practitioners in a range of settings across 20 pilot sites. They adopted an American definition for nurse practitioners: nurses with additional knowledge, skills and attitudes, who assume responsibility for health assessment and the management and delivery of services at the first level of a health care system (Bliss and Cohen, 1977). Acknowledging that many nurses working in primary care in the UK already operate in a role close to this, they also emphasized two further aspects of the style of working of their nurse practitioners: the responsibility for seeing medically unscreened patients, and discretion to diagnose, refer and treat patients across a wide range of disorders.

It emerged in the course of the project that nurse practitioners at eight out of the 20 sites did not conform to this role definition either because they were seeing patients from particular client groups (for example patients with psychiatric conditions) or because the setting (for example, based in a retail chemist shop) meant that patients mainly presented with very minor symptoms.

The project found that the nurse practitioners working within a general practice setting, rather than outside it, were more likely to operate to the full range of their skills. Patients valued the consultation styles and additional dimensions of the consultation offered by the project nurse practitioners. Independent clinical assessors found that the nurses practised safely and effectively. The two most experienced nurse practitioners tended to work more like GPs, with shorter consultation times than other nurse practitioners and less reported emphasis on the preventive aspects of the consultation, without reducing patient satisfaction noticeably. These two nurse practitioners practised in a way which reduced some elements of the cost of care. All the nurse practitioners met a 'care gap', that is, they were meeting a currently unmet need.

The authors of the evaluation commissioned by the NHS Executive concluded that any planned development of primary care should establish clearly the care gap that the development is intended to fill. In many practices the main care gap might be that patients do not feel that GPs spend enough time with them or broaden out consultations appropriately. Nurse practitioners can fill this gap within a general assessment consultation and offer the added advantage of relieving the GPs of some routine consultations. This role may be most valuable in small and single-handed practices. Often the gap may be filled most easily by developing the skills of an existing member of the primary health care team. Filling care gaps through nurse practitioner deployment in settings where there are no alternative services will necessarily increase costs. This cost should be judged relative to the care gap filled and not in isolation.

The authors further argue that there is a tension between the generic and national standard model of a nurse practitioner established in a course curriculum and qualification and the need for the role to evolve and the nurse practitioner to integrate into local primary care. They suggest that agreed national standards should be complemented by a framework for the local customization of roles to meet particular local needs. Further nurse practitioner pilots would benefit from a focus on the development of broad guidelines for the role, with local flexibility to match that role with key needs and other skills in the care team, and from the provision of a secure environment within which safety and efficiency of care are monitored while the nurse practitioner role is allowed to develop (Touche Ross, 1994).

The doctor substitute

Experience from North America and the UK suggests a number of alternative nurse practitioner models. The first is the oldest, the doctor substitute. This model fills the gaps in health care provision when medical cover is absent. This was the situation in Colorado in the early 1960s which led to the first nurse practitioners in the US being employed and still appears to be the case in remote rural areas of the US. The feldscher in Russia and barefoot doctors in China also fulfil this role. In Russia and China, economic necessity has forced the development of health workers with basic medical training, educated to deal with common ailments and with an ability to work closely with rural populations. These roles have limited applicability in the UK, which is small, densely populated and at a different stage of economic development. Not all groups have access to primary medical care, however. In this country, Burke-Masters was a doctor substitute in the 1980s for homeless alcoholics in London's East End who were not registered with a GP.

A variant of this model is the doctor substitute for emergency and first aid services, sometimes from the nursing profession but sometimes a paramedic. This function includes the personnel on UK ambulances, who provide treatment as well as transport, and also the skoraya pomoshch feldschers in Russia. The triage nurses within UK accident and emergency departments provide a non-medical first point of contact in acute situations; some nurses within accident and emergency departments also provide treatment, call for X rays and arrange discharge.

The doctor substitute model has developed in countries with a history of doctor shortages. Because of adequate medical coverage in the UK, this model has, until the 1990s, only emerged to serve groups who have difficulty in gaining access to a family doctor, for example homeless people and those suffering from chronic alcoholism. The doctor substitute model has been mooted recently in the UK to overcome medical manpower difficulties; within the hospital sector there has been a concern about junior doctors' hours, and nurses have been proposed as a substitute to do some of the doctors' work. There has been a concern about vacant junior doctor posts in accident and emergency, and the Chief Medical Officer has issued guidance to allow nurses to take on some medical work.

In Salisbury a single-area trial of nurses replacing family doctors as a first point of contact during the out-of-hours periods began in 1996. Nurses are now used in some areas in the North West Region for telephone triage to take the calls made to out-of-hours centres. Some practices are introducing nurse triage to sift the requests for 'same day' surgery appointments, the so-called 'urgent extras'. *The New NHS* White Paper includes provision for a 24-hour telephone advice line staffed by nurses, covering the whole country by the year 2000. A trend can be detected that indicates a blurring of roles, and that some substitution may be acceptable. A nurse-led primary care-led NHS would deny the public the right of direct access to a family doctor and would relegate the medical profession to a supporting role in primary care. Despite the fact that at least one Primary Care Act pilot (in Derbyshire) is exploring this avenue, a review of the literature suggests that neither the public nor the doctors are ready for this, although some limited substitution because of lack of time available or manpower difficulties may be acceptable.

The doctor's assistant

A second model is that of doctor's assistant, taking referrals from the doctor and practising within protocols in an extended nursing role. Some American nurse practitioners work in this way, particularly those specializing with a specific client group. In this country the rheumatology nurse practitioners are an example, and it could be argued that practice nursing is moving in this direction, with their developing expertise in specific chronic illness, such as asthma and diabetes.

There is evidence that this model already operates within the UK, both within primary care in the shape of practice nurses, and in the hospital sector, with the development of clinical nurse specialists and accident and emergency nurse practitioners. It fits well in primary care, since practice nurses are employed by the doctors with whom they work. But there is also evidence that nurses wish to work more autonomously than before, their desires facilitated by the issuing of the Scope of Professional Practice, the new Project 2000 nurse education system, and the role model of the autonomously practising midwife. The doctor's assistant model would ultimately be constraining to the realization of that aim.

The nurse as one half of the 'illness care: health care' dyad

A third model is that of complementing the doctor's work, providing health care where the doctor concentrates on illness care: the 'illness care: health care' dyad. In practice, this means a focus on screening, promotion and prevention work. Many Canadian nurse practitioners work in this way, and in the UK some of Barbara Stilwell's work and Monica Tettersell's work in the 1980s was along these lines. Community midwifery in the UK has also developed in this direction, with much of the routine antenatal care now provided by the midwife, with the GP or hospital obstetrician in the background for support and reassurance, and when something goes wrong. UK health visitors also carry out health prevention work.

This model presupposes that patients come with either an 'illness' for the doctor or a 'health care problem' for the nurse. The reality is, of course, more complex, with individuals often presenting problems across the range, from acute illness to health queries, particularly in first-point-of-contact care. There is evidence, however, that some patients do differentiate between medical and nursing care in this way, for example, in maternity, where some women have described the role of the midwife as giving health advice and the doctor as treating illness (Chambers, 1995). There is also an argument that nursing and medical education differs along these lines, with the latter focusing much more strongly on pathology. There may be mileage therefore in acknowledging the existence of the 'illness care: health care' dyad, while not building a nurse practitioner model entirely on this foundation.

The nurse as alternative first point of contact

A fourth model allows the public to go to the nurse as an *alternative* first point of contact to the doctor, and gives the nurse the authority for examination, diagnosis and treatment for minor complaints, following protocols agreed with the doctors, where appropriate, as well as utilizing a holistic nursing model of care. Stilwell and Restall worked successfully in this way in the 1980s, Kaufman and many others in the 1990s, and the RCN training course promotes this model (Stilwell, 1988; Kaufman, 1996). This pathway to primary health care offers patients the choice of seeing a doctor or seeing a nurse. Midwives are also used as an alternative first-point-of-contact with a query in pregnancy; these health workers are increasingly considered to be the experts in maternity care and are used for first-point-of-contact care and treatment, for queries from clients and also for straightforward deliveries.

The predominant features of this model of the nurse practitioner as an *alternative* first point of contact for primary health care are likely to be the most appropriate for the UK primary health care environment, where there has been no overall shortage of doctors (although concern on this issue is recurrently expressed), teamwork in primary health care is being encouraged and where nurses are increasingly rejecting the handmaiden role. It conforms with the current public expectation for direct access to their family doctor, while allowing patients to see an alternative practitioner if they do not want treatment which utilizes a predominantly medical approach. It also allows nurses and doctors to work together as a team, focusing on their strengths and permitting them to develop special interests and areas of particular expertise, rather than operating independently of each other. As we will see later, this is likely to be more acceptable to the two professions. The model of alternative first-point-of-contact nurse practitioner would be enhanced, however, by borrowing from the other models described above. From the first model we have seen that a measure of substitution is likely to be feasible: for example, nurse practitioner appointments may be available when doctors' appointments are fully booked. From the second model we have seen that working to some extent as a doctor's assistant builds on the present fruitful relationship which has developed between practice nurses and family doctors. From the third model the professional curricula and the patients' perspective do suggest that nurses are more geared to a health promotion and advice focus while doctors are more geared to a disease treatment focus.

Having established the most appropriate model for the UK, the next issues to address are, first, how acceptable is the nurse as an alternative first point of contact to the professions, and, second, how far is the government likely to give its blessing to this way forward for primary care?

Medical views: are nurse practitioners necessary and are they a threat?

A major piece of research into delegation in general practice was carried out by Bowling (Bowling, 1981). Her main contention is that family doctors need a clearer definition of their role before they will feel able to delegate. Bowling's survey of doctors showed that only one quarter were in favour of a nurse carrying out the initial consultation in the surgery, the main advantage being seen as a saving of the doctor's time. Of those opposed to the idea, reasons given included the complexity of diagnosis in general practice, the barrier to the doctor–patient relationship which would be created, and the role threat – some did not see a *need* for a nurse in this role. Bowling argues that this hostility stems from the fact that one of the few clearly defined aspects of the GP's role is as professional of first contact. Interestingly, a higher proportion of doctors were in favour of nurses carrying out initial home visits. The sophistication of practice organization, the range of medical activities carried out by the partners, and the recency of graduation did have a bearing on the amount of delegation practised and doctors' attitudes towards delegation. It is therefore possible that a later generation of doctors would give more favourable views.

Miller and Backett, in a larger sample than Bowling's, report a more positive attitude on the part of GPs towards the appropriateness of nurses undertaking, after suitable training, certain clinical tasks, including history taking, examination, diagnosis and advice on treatment (Miller and Backett, 1980). Two thirds were in favour of the extended role, and the characteristics most significantly associated with this new role were doctors under 50 years and practices in which regular formal meetings took place between doctors, nurses and other practice staff. This again suggests that as the older, less favourably inclined doctors retire, a greater proportion of the remaining doctor population will be interested in the new concept.

The Royal College of General Practitioners (RCGP) has approved the notion of nurse practitioners, but has called for clearly defined jobs which do not overlap with practice nurses' responsibilities, and the need for nurse practitioners to work within prmary health care teams. The RCGP has said that it would welcome experiments with nurses doing a degree of prescribing. The British Medical Association (BMA) has also expressed support for an extended role for appropriately trained nurses and sees the development of nurse practitioners as particularly desirable in extending the range of services provided within a practice (Warden, 1988). Individual doctors have, however, expressed significant reservations. It is perhaps not surprising that Barbara Burke-Masters' stand-alone model caused so much hostility among GPs, since not only was she indicating that her work was on a level with theirs, but that her presence meant that the patients could make do without a GP altogether. Stilwell's work has also generated criticism from doctors. One senior medical academic in general practice, commenting on the Stilwell experiment in the early 1980s, went so far as to say that the nurse practitioner concept in the UK was unnecessary (because there was an adequate supply of doctors), dangerous (because nurses were ill equipped to make safe diagnoses) and destructive (because the nurse practitioners would remove the GPs' continuing and personal relationship with patients (Sharron, 1984). Medical colleagues at the Birmingham University Department of General Practice who evaluated Stilwell's work with her reached more favourable conclusions (Stilwell *et al.*, 1987).

A sea change can be detected in professional opinion from the late 1980s. A survey undertaken in 1990 about GPs' attitudes towards practice nurses found that 90% of respondents wanted a further expansion of the practice nurse role and 94% felt that patients should be able to refer themselves directly to a nurse. There was a limit to this liberalization of attitudes, however: only 30% were in favour of practice nurses as independent practitioners (Robinson, Beaton and White, 1993). Then in 1991 the doctors' professional body made a surprising suggestion that the GP's traditional gatekeeping and first-point-of-contact roles could be reduced in return for a more precise definition of general medical services and a more satisfactory system of remuneration (General Medical Services Committee, 1991). Looking at primary health care from an international perspective, Fry and Horder welcome the desire of nurses to take on greater responsibilities, because there is more than enough work for both (Fry and Horder, 1994). There is a caveat and warning to goverment health policy-makers, however, not to use nurses for economic reasons, substituting workers with less appropriate training for those with more, when this would be to the disadvantage of patients.

The argument here is, broadly speaking, a workload question and, from an international perspective, this may suggest that the Alma Ata declaration (WHO, 1978), with its dominant themes about a primary care-based health service, may at last be taking some effect, although this sea change in opinion in the UK may have pragmatic origins. It can at least partially be traced to the impact of aspects of recent government health policy, including increased stress and a growing resentment with the burdens imposed by the new contract (described, for example, by Rout and Rout (1993) and Chambers and Belcher (1993)), the effects on GP workload of fundholding and other purchasing or commissioning responsibilities, and the rise in patients' expectations following the Patient's Charter.

On a more positive note, there is now a clear trend towards accepting, if not wholeheartedly welcoming, the team approach rather than working in isolation in general practice (RCGP, 1996). There is also a growing acknowledgement of the development of the nursing role within the primary health care team in order to cope with the challenges of delivering primary care in the 1990s, although there are also a host of concomitant concerns:

> ...a change in the traditional doctor–patient relationship is occurring with medical continuity of care gradually becoming displaced by nurse-led continuity for health promotion and chronic disease care and incentives being provided to doctors for a culture of delegation and teamwork rather than doing ... the balance between personal availability to the public and teamwork is an important matter because additional medical generalist manpower is not yet being planned as part of the British experiment in health service re-organisation ... the challenge in the new general practice is how to achieve the benefits of delegation without exposing patients to unreasonable risk...' (RCGP, 1996)

The conclusion must be that doctors are now considering the potential of the nursing contribution, not on a wave of altruism or as a result of a new professional laissez-faire policy, but as a survival tactic.

Nursing views: is it still nursing?

If the doctors are equivocal about the concept, how ready are nurses to contemplate pursuing this development of their nursing role? Almost two decades ago, Bowling found that the nurses were no more keen than the doctors to accept the delegation of clinical tasks (Bowling, 1981). There is concern that the acceptance of delegated tasks would diminish the 'essence' of nursing, and would divide the profession, already insecure about its status and the extent of its autonomy. However, when the Royal College of Nursing (RCN) gave evidence to the Social Services Select Committee in 1988, they declared themselves in favour of the role of nurse practitioner, as long as it was not seen as a doctor substitute. The RCN asserted that nursing in primary care was a complementary service which could be very much cheaper and better than if the same kind of service was provided by doctors (Warden, 1988). Perhaps significantly, the first nurse practitioner courses to be established in this country have been organized, in Manchester and in London, by the RCN. The first student intake was in January 1991.

There has been little research on the attitude of nurses themselves to the idea of the nurse practitioner. Practice nurses have expressed frustration with the limits to their jobs and interest in developing their role (Bowling and Stilwell, 1988). Anecdotal evidence suggests that many nurses leave the profession because they expected more responsibility, and because they felt that they were not meeting patients' psychological as well as physiological needs (Annandale-Steiner, 1979). The recession in the late 1980s may have averted the anticipated nurse shortages that had been foretold, but an analysis of the nursing manpower picture in 1996 by Buchan suggests that nursing shortages will again feature in the NHS, although they are more likely to be in the acute rather than the primary health care sector. Buchan also argues that a long-term view of nurse workforce planning should take into account not only numbers in nursing, but what motivates people to enter and to continue in nursing (Buchan, 1996).

The major driving force for change in recent years within nursing has been the issuing of the Scope of Professional Practice by the profession's regulatory body. This has liberated nursing, particularly within primary care, because it emphasizes that extended roles should no longer be legitimized by certificates, but by satisfying the principles of the Code of Professional Conduct, in particular the requirement to base nursing practice on patient needs and on the extent of the nurse's competence (UKCC, 1992). From an academic nursing perspective, Butterworth suggests that there is a case to be made for 'setting our own professional house in order' before asking for a public endorsement of the nurse practitioner role. In particular, he argues for three developments: first, that there should be safe practice through education, skill development and clinical supervision; second, articulation of practice activities; and third, individual responsibility for extended action (Butterworth, 1991). It could be argued that these are essential prerequisites for the development of nurse practitioners, but desirable and not essential for all nurses. For example, articulation of practice activities suggests a level of presentational skills to a multidisciplinary audience to which not all nurses would wish to aspire. Stilwell, from her perspective as nurse practitioner 'pioneer', concurs with Butterworth's point about safe practice but, less cautiously, also suggests that a decision on whether to proceed should only further depend on the acceptability of an extended/expanded role to patients and to colleagues (Stilwell, 1988). The question of how acceptable the nurse practitioner role is to patients and to professional colleagues is indeed crucial, as there is no point in pursuing this route if the criterion of acceptability cannot be satisfied.

In summary, therefore, it appears that the climate of opinion within the two professions may be favourably inclined towards experimentation with the notion of a nurse practitioner role, although the nurse as substitute for the doctor would clearly be unacceptable to both. There is a high degree of acceptance of the role of the specialist nurse practitioner; role conflict appears minimal with the nurse concentrating on specialist, and often very technical, *nursing* care. The more common term for this kind of post is clinical nurse specialist, but the role operates only partially as a part of the primary health care network, at least in the UK, since referrals are the norm. That leaves two further possible roles; the one that focuses on health promotion would probably be increasingly seen as already within the province of the practice nurse, particularly with her new tasks running the chronic illness clinics, the well-women and well-men clinics and carrying out the mini-medicals, in order for the doctors to fulfil the terms of their contract. The final possible role is the one in which minor illness is managed. The professions have indicated some willingness to experiment with this idea. A further assumption, however, is that current government policy on the NHS is favourably inclined towards the development of the nurse practitioner role.

Government policy: benign neglect

In 1968 the Royal Commission on Medical Education stated that GPs should be freed from routine trivial work not requiring their level of skill and expertise. In the 1970s, GPs began to work much more with practice nurses, and the number of attached community nursing staff also increased. The Cumberlege Report in 1986 recommended that the subsidy for practice nurses should be abolished (effectively encouraging their demise), that neighbourhood nursing teams should be established and concluded that the principle of introducing the nurse practitioner into primary care should be adopted. The report decided that the nurse practitioner's key tasks would be to interview patients and diagnose and treat specific diseases in accordance with the agreed medical protocols; refer to the GP patients who have medical problems which lie outside the written protocols; be available for all patients who wish to consult the nurse practitioner; give counselling and nursing advice to patients consulting her direct or referred to her by a doctor; conduct screening programmes among specific age or client groups; maintain patient care programmes, particularly to the chronic sick; and refer patients for further care to the neighbourhood nursing service (DHSS, 1986). In its response to the report, the DHSS dismissed the idea of withdrawing the practice nurse subsidy, saw some merits in the neighbourhood nursing concept, and cautiously approved the increasing interest shown in the potential for nurse practitioners, in particular in the notion that nurse practitioners could provide patients with an alternative source of initial advice. The DHSS added that 'The precise tasks would need to be worked out carefully within the practice team, and could involve both practice nurses and community nursing staff employed by health authorities' (DHSS, 1987).

There was also new guidance on *The Extending Role of the Nurse* (PL/CNO(89)10). This was contained in a working party report, which offered an updated interpretation of the health circular on the subject issued in

1977 (HC (77) 22). The original circular recognized that in both primary and specialist health care, nurses had become increasingly involved in tasks, procedures and decision making, which had previously been a medical responsibility. Although the remit of the working party which reinterpreted the circular excluded nurses employed by GPs, their report suggests that the principles recommended in the updated guidance are equally relevant to this group of nurses. The main points in the 1987 guidance were:

- a definition of the extending role: '... activities normally undertaken by doctors but which may be delegated in appropriate circumstances, and which may be performed by nurses with appropriate training and competence'

- extending the nurse's role remains crucial to the provision and development of patient care

- there is no consensus within the professions nationally as to which tasks fall appropriately within the nurse's extending role

- the legal implications of extending roles require more careful scrutiny

- role extension should not be at the expense of the performance of the nurse's customary activities

- activities within the extended role should be recognized by the professions, although a national list of specific activities would not be practicable, and would militate against the development of methods of working which are appropriate in some local circumstances but not in others

- the nurse must be specifically and adequately trained for the particular delegated activities.

Perhaps the two most interesting issues in this guidance were: first, the government's intention that the nurse's role must, in the interest of patient care, continue to develop and, second, the apparent support for locally based innovative projects that do not necessarily require national professional endorsement.

The other initiative has been in the area of nurse prescribing. This was an area in which Cumberlege had recommended improvements, because in practice, in the community, a doctor often 'rubber stamps' a prescribing decision taken by a nurse. This can lead to a lack of clarity about professional relationships and, added Cumberlege, is demeaning to both doctors and nurses. The report of the Advisory Group on Nurse Prescribing in 1989 recommended that suitably qualified nurses working in the community should be able to prescribe from a limited list of items, including some drugs which are available over the counter and some prescription-only medicines (POMs). The report suggested that there could be significant benefit to patient care if nurses were able to provide rapid treatment of minor infections. In addition, nurse prescribing would make more effective use of nurses' training and skills, with work being carried out at the most appropriate professional level. This in turn would enable the best use to be made of the time and skills of other professionals in the team. The report was issued for comment by the government, and responses were generally favourable and supportive of its recommendations. The government declared its support, in principle, for nurse prescribing but delayed implementation, pending an independent cost benefit analysis of the advisory group's proposals. Pilot schemes are now under way assessing the impact of nurse prescribing from a limited list of drugs. This list is indeed so limited as to be deemed derisory by many nurses. The government's support for nurse prescribing must therefore be interpreted as only lukewarm, in view of the speed with which much more fundamental NHS reforms have been implemented.

Following the Cumberlege Report, the reports on the extending role and on nurse prescribing, there were two White Papers, followed by the NHS and Community Care Act 1990, signalling fundamental changes in the way the NHS was to be run. In addition, a new GP contract establishing tighter control and setting higher standards for primary medical care was implemented in April 1990. It is therefore perhaps not surprising that there was little more said on the nurse practitioner issue, particularly in the general practice setting, during that period.

Following the bedding down of the early 1990s NHS reforms, a 'listening exercise' started by ministers in 1995 to identify a way forward for primary care led to a fresh description of the role of nurse practitioners in primary care, in which the nurse practises autonomously, manages a complete episode of care and may be responsible for people who have not already been seen by a GP; this was hailed as 'an important new development' (NHSE, 1996), but there was also a warning that there needed to be changes in the way primary health care teams work if nurses are to develop greater clinical autonomy. A lead from the centre is not at hand: '...the pace at which these kind of developments take place are for local decision but the centre could also explore ways of encouraging such developments and removing the barriers to them, for example by considering whether there should be a widening of the ability of different professional groups to prescribe ... medicines or a more practice based approach to the GP contract which could explicitly take into account the role and contribution of different professionals...' (ibid). The Primary Care Act of 1997 does indeed allow for new models of the GP contract to be explored, and some of the pilots being funded as a result of the Act, which are due to go live in April 1998, are exploring new roles for nurses within experimental contractual frameworks, including one nurse-led family practice in Derbyshire. There is no mention of the nurse practitioner role in *The New NHS* White Paper as an alternative first point of contact at the surgery, other than in the envisaged role for nurses in manning the telephones on the NHS Direct 24-hour helpline.

It appears that the government is favourably inclined to the idea of the nurse practitioner, and local initiatives would receive support, but the details of how to proceed, with national guidance, have not been worked out. It may be seen as a 'professional' question, and details have been left on the professional advisers' desks in Leeds for endless debate and little agreement with the profession's representatives. There is therefore no push from the centre, and there are conflicting messages from the professions, but there is no opposition movement and there does appear to be a groundswell of support for the idea from some nurses and doctors, and from patients.

Evolution of a suitable and sustainable model

The nurse practitioner model which is proposed for detailed scrutiny in this book draws mainly from the one which has the nurse as alternative first point of contact for patients in primary care. This professional is:

- an experienced nurse with appropriate additional qualifications who offers primary health care consultations on undifferentiated health problems as an alternative first point of contact to going to see the family doctor

- a nurse to whom patients can go for diagnosis, treatment and advice for minor illness and for other health matters which patients may consider are appropriate for a nurse consultation

- a member of the primary health care team who works closely with other colleagues, especially the family doctor, and whose work is guided but not bound by protocols

- a nurse who largely focuses on a holistic nursing approach to health care but who draws from the medical model of health and illness where appropriate.

The Derbyshire Project

The model described above was chosen as the cornerstone of a project to examine the impact of introducing nurse practitioners into general practice by Derbyshire FHSA. The plan was to utilize nursing skills more fully, enable GPs to practise their medical skills more extensively and give greater choice to patients. The aim was not to develop a doctor substitute, and direct access for patients to their GP would not be affected. The project would assess the potential impact of the nurse practitioner on the quality of care provided in the practice setting and on the sense of job satisfaction for the nurses and doctors in the primary health care team, thereby addressing the issues of desirability, acceptability and practicability of the nurse practitioner concept in primary health care.

Out of 19 who initially expressed interest, three volunteer practices in Derbyshire were chosen to take part in the project. A common job description for the part-time nurse practitioner role was drawn up for use. The nurse practitioner was to focus on providing an alternative surgery consultation service for patients, working closely with GPs and other members of the primary health care team. Her workload would encompass the diagnosis and treatment of minor illness, and general health advice and information. Patients would have a choice of consulting with either one of the doctors or the nurse practitioner. Funding was made available for the three part-time grade H posts (ten hours per week) at 100% level of reimbursement by the FHSA for two years. A training allowance was also made available to purchase relevant off-the-shelf courses and to take up other training opportunities as they arose. The reason for the generous reimbursement level was the substantial time commitment, in training terms, which would be required by each practice, and uncertainty about potential benefits. Management of the project was provided by an independent project coordinator-evaluator with support from FHSA staff. For the purposes of evaluation, three control practices were chosen which had similar features and served similar populations as the participating practices.

The three volunteer Derbyshire practices had broadly similar characteristics, serving a mixture of suburban and semi-rural populations, and each having one woman partner or assistant. The Ongar Practice (all names have been changed) appointed a nurse practitioner in 1990, as an additional member of staff, who was recruited for 15 hours a week (ten hours paid under the nurse practitioner scheme). This nurse practitioner trained intensively for two months and started her own surgeries in December 1990. Her background is in hospital nursing and midwifery. This is a fundholding practice in the north of the county in an industrial/marketing town whose working population largely commute into Manchester. For historical reasons the practice has a higher-than-expected number of women patients on its list. The surgery is situated in a purpose-built building and had three partners, one of whom was a woman, until August 1992, when a fourth partner joined the practice. By the end of 1997 the same nurse was still in post: she had taken a nurse practitioner diploma qualification at Manchester University (a qualification not available at the time the project was in progress). Her hours had been increased from 15 to 30, at H grade, and eight of those were to discharge management responsibilities for health promotion and as first line manager for the practice nurses. Her clinical workload still focuses on minor illness, children and women's health, her surgeries are very popular and she reports that she still enjoys the work!

The Johns Practice appointed an existing experienced practice nurse with a background in health visiting to the post in November 1990, on the basis that ten hours would be 'ringfenced' for nurse practitioner consulting time. This nurse started her own surgeries in March 1991. This is a rural fundholding and training practice of four male partners covering three Derbyshire villages with a purpose-built centre and two branch surgeries. There is also a permanent woman GP assistant employed by the practice. By the end of 1997 this nurse was still in post, and still running nurse practitioner surgeries. The main development was that she and the senior district nurse are now first on-call for the practice once a week for 12 hours from midday to midnight. In the first year of operation, 60% of calls were resolved by advice giving without needing to contact the duty doctor.

The Sanders Practice appointed an existing practice nurse with a background in midwifery, who had been based at the branch surgery for the previous two years, to the post of nurse practitioner in January 1991. The nurse began her own surgeries at the branch working alongside one of the GPs in April 1991. This is an urban practice with its branch surgery in the middle of a large privately owned housing estate on the edge of town. Two years later the nurse moved to work with another practice in Derbyshire to develop their practice nursing services; after six months she started to work alongside the doctors as an alternative first point of contact for patients, including for minor injuries work, which the practice experienced significant demand for, the nearest casualty department being some seven miles away. A change in personal circumstances a year later necessitated a move to Scotland.

At the start of the project there were no externally organized nurse practitioner courses available. Each nurse, with support from the FHSA, identified her training needs in order to comfortably and safely take up her new position as an alternative point of first contact for patients. The seven methods of training used are outlined in Box 2.1. Each practice nominated a GP mentor to guide and advise the nurse. This doctor also planned and managed the practice-based training programme in conjunction with the nurse. The GP mentor notion was later to be adopted in the RCN nurse practitioner diploma course.

Box 2.1   Derbyshire Nurse Practitioner Project: methods of training

1 Sitting in on GP consultations to enhance practical skills of examination, history taking, diagnosis and treatment

2 Private study extending knowledge of anatomy and physiology

3 Tutorials with the FHSA pharmacy facilitator on pharmacology

4 Observing consultant outpatient clinics

5 Liaison with other specialists in the field

6 Attendance at relevant courses to bridge skill gaps

Training for the new role was always recognized as continuous and opportunities were identified throughout the project. These included commissioning Barbara Stilwell to carry out a two-day assessment with a focus on identifying further training needs, an invitation to a United Kingdom Central Council (UKCC) officer to debate and clarify attitudes of senior representatives of the profession towards nurse practitioners, and attendance at the American Nurse Practitioner Conference in Colorado, USA, the 'birthplace' in the 1960s of the nurse practitioner concept.

What the patients, nurses and doctors in these three practices thought about the new nurse practitioner service is described in the following chapters. Their experiences are also compared with others in the UK to determine the potential future for the expansion of this model.

3

The consultation experience

What do patients think about nurse practitioners? In the Derbyshire Nurse Practitioner Project postal questionnaires were sent twice to the three volunteer practices and to the three matched control practices – once before the nurse practitioner started surgeries and then 18 months later. A total of 2400 questionnaires were mailed and, with one reminder, a response rate of 76% was achieved. A copy of the questions asked in the patients' questionnaire and correspondence with the hypotheses under test is provided in Appendix A. A series of six focus groups with the primary health care teams was held to probe the perspectives of the nurses and doctors on the nurse practitioner role. A fuller account of the research methods employed is available elsewhere (Chambers, 1996b).

More choice for patients

The figures indicate a reasonable depth of penetration by the nurse practitioners into the population of the research practices over the period of 18 months, particularly in view of the fact that they were providing only 10 surgery consultation hours per week. Respondents in the volunteer practices were asked how often they had consulted with the nurse practitioner. Nineteen per cent had consulted her once, a further 20% had consulted her 2–4 times and 4% had consulted her between five and nine times. Of those who had consulted a nurse practitioner (n = 189), 110 were women, 28 were parents consulting for their children and 51 were men. This compares with 77 women, 49 parents for their children and 68 men who had consulted the GP at least once, but not the nurse practitioner.

This suggests a degree of acceptability which does not appear to come from the nurse acting as a doctor substitute, since access to doctor appointments was already good: over 60% reported being able to get a doctor's appointment for a non-urgent health problem within 24 hours. It also suggests that the nurse practitioner option was more popular for women than it was for men.

The structured questions in this survey did not tackle the issue of *why* these respondents chose to consult the nurse practitioner or why, in the case of those who had seen her more than once, they chose to go back to her. Some clues are available. It is clear that these respondents liked the nurse practitioner's style of consultation from the satisfaction scores that were achieved (this is described in more detail later in this chapter). A measure of the nurse practitioner's acceptability is also apparent from the few additional comments specifically about the nurse practitioner offered at the end of the questionnaires:

> ...nurse practitioner system better for patient and doctor...
> ...prefer the nurse practitioner, because there all the time... [the Sanders practice where the nurse practitioner provided consultations at the branch surgery]
> ...nurse practitioner is excellent...
> ...nurse more friendly and caring than the doctors especially where children are concerned...

Further information about why patients might choose to see a nurse practitioner does emerge from a later study conducted with the Johns Practice (Chambers, 1995a), the aim of which was to identify what patients considered to be the important features of all the nursing services provided from the practice (including health visiting and midwifery) and where they perceived the strengths and weaknesses lay. The method chosen to elicit this information was a combination of focus groups and single depth interviews. The nurse practitioner role was debated in all five focus groups, and was of particular interest to the women under 65. Four main sets of views emerged. First, some participants had had experience of the nurse practitioner, and expressed confidence in the service, for various reasons: because the nurse '...seemed to know what she was talking about...', the receptionists would not offer her if she was not appropriate, and she called a doctor in if she was not sure about something. One woman said that, when making an appointment, she asked for the nurse practitioner rather than the doctor '...if I feel it is something she can cope with: I find her very good...'. A second strand of opinion was that it was a worthwhile role, particularly to relieve pressure on the doctors. A third view expressed by some participants was that the role was unknown to them but they were interested in finding out more, particularly how she could be consulted as a first point of contact and what the arrangements for prescribing were. Fourth, there were some more wary participants who wanted more information about the role and a reassurance that the nurse had been appropriately trained. They described how their notion about a nurse's role did not fit with what they recently experienced or were discussing in the focus group:

> ...Why do they put you in to see her when she is not a qualified doctor? I don't know what her qualifications are ... my experience with [the nurse] is in the family planning clinic and with my blood pressure ... and then I came for

my ear or something and I thought: what is she looking in my ear for? ...
you've got an image of what a nurse does and you think that she is not qualified to diagnose anything else...

...we are not given enough information ... when you think of a doctor, you
know that they have been through all those years of training ... but if they
gave us more information on what a nurse could do...

The 1995 study suggests that having trust in the nurse's professional standards of care is an important factor in the patient's decision to choose to
see her, and not having that trust, because of a certain view about what
nurses 'do', and in the absence of other information, can be a barrier.
Some patients develop trust according to outdated role models in nursing
and will take time to adjust to the fact that nurses have moved on and
acquired more skills. In a review of women's attitudes to nurses, health
visitors and midwives, Miles also found that there was widespread confusion about which profession nurses belong to and the precise nature of
their expertise (Miles, 1991).

There is an interesting comparison with the theme that emerged in the
focus group discussions with the participating practice teams about the
level of trust which doctors place in nurses. Not only some patients, but
some doctors are doubtful about whether they can put trust in nurses
working in this way. What does seem to emerge from this research, the
study of nursing services in the Johns Practice and earlier American
studies is that experience of, in comparison with the notion of, a nurse
practitioner service increases its acceptability to patients and doctors.

An opportunity to consult with someone of the same gender

It emerged from the focus group discussions in the Derbyshire research
that the primary health care teams saw the nurse as providing additional
surgery appointment times for patients to meet growing demands, the
choice of a more relaxed consultation with a lesser likelihood of a
prescription as an outcome and the choice of another woman practitioner.
(In each of these three practices, there was only one part-time woman
doctor.)

How important is the personal relationship with nurses in general? The
structured questions did not address this issue, but there were a few
comments volunteered by the respondents at the end of the questionnaire.
One respondent valued the continuity of care provided by her health
visitor, and several mentioned the value of the midwife in providing

comprehensive antenatal care. Most comments about the nurse practitioner came from respondents registered at the branch surgery where the nurse had a high profile. They liked being able to go and see her because they knew she was there all the time, whereas there were always different doctors. They also liked going to see her because she was a woman.

In the focus groups the nurse practitioners mentioned their value, in patients' eyes, because they were female and (in two out of three cases) parents of young children. There was a suggestion that the relationship was potentially closer because there was less of a social difference between nurse and patient than between doctor and patient, and that this closeness was in some circumstances welcomed by patients. The nurse practitioner at the branch surgery mentioned that she felt that patients had developed a growing trust and confidence in her as they got to know her. Patients positively chose, and appeared to appreciate contact with, someone who could speak the nurse's 'language', someone who had an understanding, perhaps through a greater overlap of common experiences, of their lives and whom they could also trust as a competent professional person. The implication here is that (in the nurse practitioners' view, at least) the patients chose to see nurse practitioners because they were likely to be able to communicate better with them than with the doctors.

In the Johns Practice, the nurse reported:

> ...quite a lot of people have come to talk to me, because they know that I can help them ... and they don't always want to talk to a doctor...

In the Sanders Practice, where the nurse worked at the branch surgery alongside a different doctor each day, she felt that patients chose to see her because:

> ...they know me so well ... especially the mothers ... and probably because of that they have built up some sort of trust in me ... they trust my opinion ... they know that if I am not sure, I will tell them I am not sure, and ask them to see the doctor...

It is difficult to disentangle whether the important fact was that the nurse practitioners were *nurses* who were also women from a closer social background to the patients than the doctors or whether woman *doctors* with similar social origins would have fulfilled the same purpose. There is evidence that women doctors are more patient centred than men doctors and that female patients receive a more patient-centred service from GPs of their own sex than from GPs of the opposite sex (Law and Britten, 1995). On the other hand, some of what the nurse practitioners said suggests that a woman who was a doctor rather than a nurse could be something of an inhibitor to patients to a satisfactory consultation for some health matters, because of their perceptions of the preciousness of the doctor's time.

The developing nurse–patient relationship

The information from this research is insufficient to draw firm conclusions about the nature and value of the nurse–patient relationship, and this particular research path is less well trodden than the one concerning the doctor–patient relationship. The evaluation of the South Thames Region pilot nurse practitioner projects did include focus groups with patients, and found from these that patients valued a more relaxed and equal style of consultation with nurse practitioners, and also felt able to take a wider range of less specific and less serious health problems (Touche Ross, 1994). In addition, the case study examining the patients' perspective of all the primary and community nursing services available at the Johns Practice provides evidence of the features in the nurse–patient relationship which patients find important. These include reliability, trust in the nurses' clinical competence and also the depth of the personal service provided, which provides some indication that patients value continuity of care from nurses as well as from their doctor. The following comment also suggests a therapeutic value to the nurse–patient relationship on a par with the flash of understanding explored by Balint in the doctor–patient relationship:

> ... They're [the nurses] all friendly; they treat you on a person to person basis ... *it's as though they know all about you.* [emphasis added] ... especially my family: they always ask how everyone else is ... they're interested in you and your family ... it's a very personal service. (Chambers, 1995a)

Miles argues that relationships with nurses are on a different plane from those with doctors: for example, nursing advice is seen as essentially common-sense lay guidance, and the nurse's practical experience is seen as more valid than the extent of her book-learning; negative patient attitudes can stem from criticism that a midwife or health visitor has had no baby of their own. Miles also comments that, as noted by the nurse practitioners described in this book, there is less of a marked social difference between the nurse and the patient than between the doctor and the patient, and women patients often emphasize that nurses are more approachable and it is easier to relax and talk to them than it is to doctors (Miles, 1991). These features of the nurse–patient relationship, together with the findings from this book, particularly on the high level of patient satisfaction with the nurse consultation, are clues to guide further research work, particularly on the question of the nurse as a health professional who is also a(nother) woman and a person who can draw on similar life experiences as the patient.

The lack of conclusive evidence is partly a reflection of the research design in the Derbyshire Project, which did not set out to explore the nurse–patient relationship, and also a consequence of the comparatively short history in surgery-based primary health care of nurses providing holistic care, rather than carrying out specific tasks delegated by doctors. Within specific client groups in primary care there is, however, evidence of a high value placed by some patients on strong personal relationships, particularly maternity patients with midwives for antenatal, intrapartum and postnatal care (Chambers, 1995b). The success of the midwife–patient relationship has led to the development of the notion of the midwife as 'lead carer', suggesting a closer relation with the midwife than with the GP. On the other hand, although there is a high level of continuity of care with health visitors, the health visitor–parent relationship is more problematic, and a model of health visitors as lead carers has not been mooted (see, for example, Mellor and Chambers, 1995). The difference in the relationships with midwives and with health visitors may be to do with differences in the degree of confidence experienced, and the extent of professional and managerial autonomy which midwives and health visitors exercise. Midwives, for example, have clinical principal status, which sets them apart legally from other nurses. Further research is required to examine what it is that patients value in their relationship with nurses and what factors lead to successful relationships between nurses and patients.

Patient-devised triage

In the Johns and Sanders Practices there were attempts to differentiate between what a nurse–patient consultation and a doctor–patient consultation might be like, and resistance to the notion that the nurse would be substituting for the doctor. In the Sanders Practice one of the doctors hoped that the nurse practitioner might 'educate' patients and therefore reduce the doctors' workload. He did not elaborate on this because the discussion then took a different turn, with a debate as to whether nurses would eventually replace many GPs because they would be cheaper. It is possible that the doctor in question may have meant by 'patient education' that the nurse would spend more, rather than less, time with patients who were consulting inappropriately and get to the nub of the problem, thereby tackling the 'revolving door' syndrome in which patients keep coming back to no benefit. In an echo of this point, doctors' increasing workloads and the issue of frequent attenders is addressed in an editorial in the *British Journal of General Practice*, and includes a suggestion that teamwork and referral within the primary health care team may not only reduce attendances, but also improve clinical care (Neal *et al.*, 1996).

In the Ongar and Sanders Practices the nurses reported that patients would go to see them *first* about a problem to find out if it was serious enough for the doctor – a kind of patient-organized triage system. The conclusion here is that the patients needed help from the nurse practitioners in categorizing their health problems*. This informal arrangement may be a vote of no confidence on the part of the patients in the formal organization. There is also an implication here that the nurse's time is somehow not as valuable as a doctor's time, and this perception is shared by both the patients and the nurse herself. In financial terms, this is probably true, given the differential in costs to train and pay doctors and nurses. The implication may go beyond financial considerations, though: according to all three teams, patients are worried about 'wasting the doctor's time'. They also 'used' the nurse practitioner (and indeed the other nursing members of the team) for clarification of their doctor's explanations of diagnoses and treatments which they had not fully understood, rather than going back to the doctor. In other words, many patients may have perceived a difference in professional and social status between their doctor and the nurse, placed a value on that difference and then chosen to see the nurse for those occasions when either professional was appropriate to meet their needs.

Predicted and unanticipated benefits

Were there differences between the professionals' *predictions* concerning the benefits to patients of the nurse practitioner role and their views *in the light of experience* of the benefits which this nurse had brought to patients? The two sets of focus group discussions provided an opportunity to highlight similarities and differences. In many areas, there was a high degree of congruence between the two; these included:

- the increase in availability of general surgery appointments
- the opportunity of a consultation without having to see the doctor
- the availability of another woman practitioner
- less pressurized consultations
- more consultations without prescriptions

---

*Triage comes from the French '*trier*' which means 'to sort'.

- more preventive health care.

In addition, in the Johns Practice one of the doctors in the team had anticipated there being a 'new professional' available for patients, who combined some new medical skills acquired from training with the doctors in the practice with nursing and counselling skills, and who would have the opportunity to practise these in a longer consultation than the doctors were able to provide. In the second focus group discussion the nurse practitioner did indeed highlight this benefit by saying that she was offering something new, she was better informed, with more skills, and was able to go further with the patient in the investigation of the health problem without referring to a doctor.

The main differences in anticipated and realized benefits were threefold:

- the availability of the nurse practitioner surgery consultation service for children for the treatment of minor illlness had not been mentioned in the first round

- the welcomed opportunity for a consultation with a health practitioner who shared a greater base of commonly shared experiences with the patient had not been foreseen

- the confusion wrought by the title 'nurse practitioner', leading to some patients thinking they were seeing a doctor and others booking in to see the practice nurse by mistake, had not been anticipated.

These differences have policy implications if this role were to be more widely marketed and implemented; this is discussed in more detail later in the book.

Had the type of work which the nurse practitioner carried out changed over time? Over the 18-month period between the first and second round of group discussions the nurse in the Ongar Practice reported a discernible swing towards carrying out consultations with a counselling component and a corresponding swing of patients seen to the 40–65 age group. During this period the nurse had gone on a counselling course and started up the practice's hormone replacement therapy (HRT) clinic. In the Johns Practice the nurse practitioner had grown generally busier, especially when one or more of the doctors was away. This nurse had also been on a basic counselling skills course, and had reorganized her workload to combine her 'nurse practitioner' surgeries and her 'practice nurse' sessions. In the Sanders Practice the nurse said that she was generally prescribing less often (about 50% of her consultations resulted in a prescription) and she was seeing more patients with asthma, in which she had developed a special interest But they were all still seeing a substantial amount of patients with gynaecological problems and patients with acute minor illness, especially children with coughs and colds.

The nurses were therefore generally seeing the same kind of health problems that came the way of the doctors, with a focus, as planned, on minor illness and women's health. What had not come out in the first round of group discussions was that, as well as becoming competent in the general run of health problems which people presented in surgery, they would also be developing special interests outside minor illness and running condition-specific clinics in addition to their surgeries. This is of course what doctors and, increasingly, practice nurses do, encouraged by the new inducements to practices in the 1990 GP contract.

In these three practices, therefore, patients were now getting a choice of GP or nurse practitioner to consult in general surgeries, and health promotion and disease management clinics run by nurses or doctors with an interest or expertise in those particular areas. From the patients' point of view there was a wider choice of health professionals with overlapping knowledge and skills. Having made their choice to see her, what did the Derbyshire Project patients think of the nurse practitioner's consultation skills?

Inside the consulting room

Respondents were asked the same questions about the quality of their consultation experience with the nurse practitioner as they had been asked about their doctor, that is, how well did they think the nurse practitioner listened, explained things, provided information and allocated time? The results for respondents who had consulted a nurse practitioner at least once are given in comparison with the doctor in Figures 3.1–3.4. Combining the consultation satisfaction rates of all three practices, the nurses score more highly than the doctors in all four aspects. The most striking difference is in the satisfaction scores for the time element in the consultation, with 178 out of 189 respondents (94%) indicating that they had enough time with the nurse practitioner, in comparison with 134 respondents (71%) indicating that they had enough time with the doctor.

The results show that the nurse practitioners were providing the respondents with a consultation experience – at least as measured by these four aspects of listening, explaining, information and time – which was better than that provided by the doctor. The difference in dissatisfaction counts was statistically significant: the null hypothesis that there was no difference between levels of dissatisfaction between patient consultations with the nurse practitioner and patient consultations with the doctor can be overturned (see Appendix B for details of results). Because of the relatively

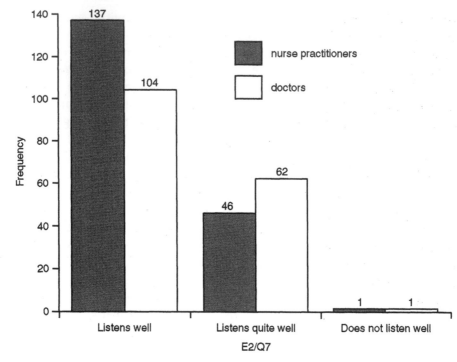

Figure 3.1   How well does the nurse practitioner/doctor listen?

small numbers involved (only 189 respondents had consulted one of the nurse practitioners), caution should be exercised in extrapolating this result to the whole population served by these three nurse practitioners.

Respondents were also asked how they would generally rate the different aspects of care given by the nurse practitioner. The results are given in Figure 3.5, which also compares these respondents' ratings given for the care given by the doctor. Fifty one (25%) rated the care given by the doctor as excellent and 72 (36%) rated the care given by the nurse practitioner as excellent. Twenty seven (13%) rated the care by the doctor as fair or poor and 15 (9%) rated the nurse practitioner care as fair or poor. These results, which again are statistically significant, provide corroboration of the findings with regard to the different dimensions of the consultation: the respondents rated the care given by the nurses more highly than the care given by the doctor.

One way of establishing the credibility of these findings is to identify how they compare with other studies of patient satisfaction with the nurse practitioner consultation. There are a number of other pieces of research on this particular question. From the US, the Office of Technology Assessment found that patients were satisfied with the care they received from nurse practitioners, and in particular they were more satisfied than with the care received from physicians in terms of 'personal care exhibited,

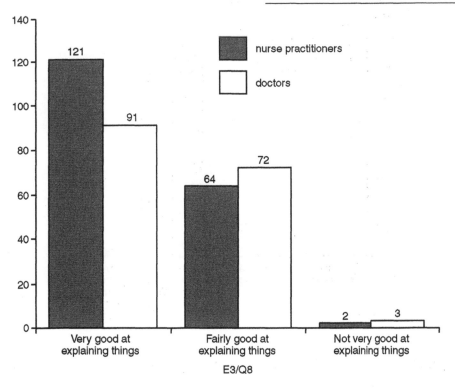

Figure 3.2   How good is the nurse practitioner/doctor at explaining things?

reduction in the professional mystique of health care delivery, amount of information conveyed, and cost of care' (Office of Technology Assessment, 1986). In the UK, Stilwell found that respondents valued the fact that the nurse was good at listening, explaining and seemed to have more time (Stilwell, 1988). Touche Ross found that 73% of patients were 'extremely satisfied' with nurse practitioners in comparison with 52% who were 'extremely satisfied' with GPs. Touche Ross also conducted focus groups with patients who had seen the nurse practitioner. The responses from these groups indicated a distinct role for nurse practitioners, meeting demands for time and sensitivity/openness which patients felt were less well met by doctors (Touche Ross, 1994).

In a single-practice study aimed at piloting a standardized patient satisfaction questionnaire, Poulton found that there were three factors associated with patient satisfaction with the nursing consultation: satisfaction with professional care, depth of the relationship and perceived time. Two separate variables were also used in a subsequent survey at the practice relating to the nurse practitioner role: acceptability of seeing the nurse practitioner instead of the doctor and avoidance of the duplication of care. The results of the survey showed overwhelming acceptance of the nurse

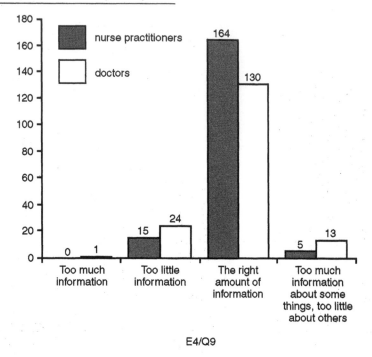

E4/Q9

Figure 3.3   How much information does the practitioner/doctor give you?

practitioner role by the patients surveyed, and high levels of satisfaction with the professional care and amount of time spent with the nurse practitioner (Poulton, 1995).

Two recurring themes running through these patient-led evaluations of the nurse practitioner style of consultation include the sense that the nurse has more time and that she has a less formal approach which facilitates a closer relationship with the patient. Both of these are important considerations for patients. The doctors and nurses in the Derbyshire Project corroborated the importance of these aspects of the consultation. They felt that the nurse was able to offer a more relaxed form of consultation and was often able to indicate and make use of shared experiences, for example, motherhood.

What is it about the nurse–patient interaction that patients value? Unconnected with this study, qualitative research conducted more recently in one of the three participating practices to obtain a patients' and carers' perspective of the whole range of primary and community nursing services found out what patients valued about nurses (Chambers, 1995a). These included the nurse practitioner and also the district nurses, practice nurse, health visitor and midwife. Patients described nursing care which was strongly focused on them as individuals as well as on their illnesses. The nurses did not allude to other pressures, concerns or other patients waiting for them. They were given time to raise their concerns. They felt valued.

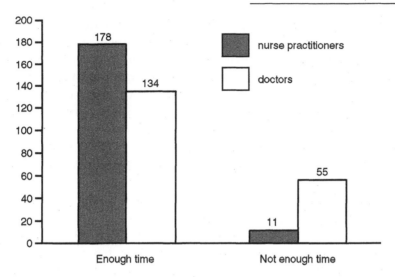

Figure 3.4   Do you have enough time with the nurse practitioner/doctor?

But patients also frequently mentioned their view that the nurses had, and applied, a high degree of technical skill in their work; the patients expected these high standards and any deviation from that did or would

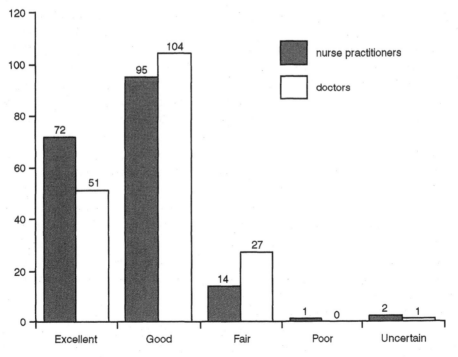

Figure 3.5   How would you describe the care you get from the nurse practitioner/doctor?

immediately alter their opinion of them. They also mentioned the organizational aspects of care which were important to them, not all of which were currently successfully being carried out. These included being able to see or otherwise contact a nurse quickly, prior warning of a home visit, home visits never being 'missed', and evidence of close teamwork and good inter-professional relations. In summary, patients from this later study identified nurses' dedication, technical skill and capacity for coordination as three key strengths. It is likely that it was these same strengths that the respondents appreciated about the nurse practitioner in the three participating practices.

Another reason for the nurses' high scores could be the length of their consultations. Although not the subject of this research, it is known that nurses tend to book longer appointments (Touche Ross, 1994), and in the three research practices the nurses tended to have ten minutes and the doctors five minutes for their surgery appointments. Within that longer time span, it is more likely that they could listen well, give adequate explanations and information, and allocate enough time.

One further point is that these results could be explained by gender difference. Most of the doctors in all three practices were men and the three nurses were women, and women are supposedly better listeners and more sensitive communicators than men. Does it matter if most doctors are men and the majority of nurses are women? The answer is that it does matter, because the current structure of primary care provides patients with a doctor, who is usually a man, as a first point of contact, whereas these results suggest that a nurse practitioner, who is usually a woman, would provide a more favourable consultation experience.

Did the gender question affect the results in the Derbyshire Project? Statistically significant differences were found in respondents' satisfaction with the GP consultation, the nurse practitioner consultation and the overall care given. The question should now be posed whether these differences are related to the case mix of patients who presented to the GP and to the nurse practitioners. Appendix C provides a separate analysis for women, children and men of the 'consultation dissatisfaction' counts and 'excellent care' counts.

Twice as many women (n = 110) as men (n = 51) had consulted the nurse practitioner as well as the GP, and the number of children presenting was half (n = 28) the number of men. Less marked differences between men (n = 68), women (n = 77) and children (n = 49) were found in the respondents who had consulted a GP at least once, but not a nurse practitioner. This would suggest that the availability of a nurse practitioner service was particularly popular for the women respondents.

Among the respondents, a statistically significant level of difference between consultation dissatisfaction counts for GPs and for nurse practitioners was found only in the women respondents, and when the totals from the three groups are aggregated. As for the numbers of respondents scoring their overall care from the GP and from the nurse practitioner as 'excellent', there are no significant differences except, again, when the totals from the three groups of respondents are combined. The numbers of men and of parents responding on behalf of their children are small, and the proportion within this small group indicating either dissatisfaction with the consultation or an excellent score for overall care is also small. This must limit the confidence which can be placed in this aspect of the findings, and indicates a focus for further work.

4 Nurse practitioners and the organization of primary care

The care gap

One of the aims of the Derbyshire Nurse Practitioner Project was to see whether an additional nurse practitioner consultation service would ease the pressure of demand for surgery appointments, reduce waiting times in the surgery and free up time for doctors to concentrate on patients with more medically complex problems while the nurses were seeing some of the patients presenting with minor illnesses.

We know that one of the aspects of the general practitioner service which patients find important is the ease of getting an appointment with the doctor. Does the presence of the nurse practitioner contributing 10 additional consulting hours to the practice make any difference to the level of accessibility to a doctor's appointment? The null hypothesis is that the nurse practitioner makes no difference to accessibility to a doctor's appointment. This was not overturned by the results (see Appendix B), which indicated very similar levels of accessibility for non-urgent appointments between the two survey rounds in each of the six practices. The only slight difference was in terms of access within 24 hours, where each of the three participating practices scored a slight increase in the proportion of respondents who said they were able to get an appointment within that period while each of the three control practices scored a slight decrease in the proportion able to be seen, but the results were not statistically significant.

Length of waiting times in the surgery were found from previous studies also to be an important feature of the quality of the service for patients. The most frequent wait beyond the appointment time was between ten and 20 minutes in both survey rounds, with 79% being seen within 30 minutes in the first survey round, rising to 82% in the second. There was no statistical difference between the length of waits for the participating practices between the first and second survey rounds so the null hypothesis cannot overturned.

No other study has addressed this question precisely, but the recent Touche Ross evaluation of the South Thames Nurse Practitioner Projects for the NHS Executive made a provisional finding that there was no tendency for the introduction of nurse practitioners to *reduce* the rate of consultation of patients, and in three project sites there was a tendency for the overall rate of consultation of all kinds to *rise* (Touche Ross, 1994). There is also evidence in the US literature (Holmes *et al.*, 1976) that consultations rise with the introduction of nurse practitioners. This would explain why patients did not record any improvements in waiting time to see a doctor. On the other hand, the slight, but not statistically significant, improvement in the Derbyshire study practices in rates of access within 24 hours for a non-urgent appointment may possibly be due to the fact that some of the 'extras' – the patients without appointments who say that they need to see a doctor urgently – are being offered the choice of seeing the nurse practitioner, thus freeing up doctor appointment spaces, which are then filled by patients with a not so urgent health problem. Indeed, some practices are now focusing on using a nurse practitioner to all intents and purposes as a doctor substitute, to meet the demand for 'urgent' or 'same day' appointments (Kaufman, 1996).

The proportions of patients who reported getting an appointment quickly in the Derbyshire Project were probably higher than is often the case elsewhere. In a comparable national study (Jacoby, 1989) only 22% of 374 patients reported being seen within 24 hours in comparison with 61% of patients in the first survey round and 63% in the second survey round in the Derbyshire Project. Twenty five per cent of the national sample reported waiting three days or longer for a non-urgent appointment, in comparison with only 11% in this research. This would suggest that the Derbyshire practices were already excellent performers, and there may have been little room for improvement. It is not known whether the null hypothesis would be overturned if the nurse practitioner role was introduced into practices where there were long waits for doctors' appointments.

In any event, the result does suggest that practices who seek to deal with pressure on surgery appointments by recruiting a nurse practitioner should proceed with caution. The presence of the nurse practitioner may enable additional patients to be seen, thus meeting a 'care gap', but demand to see the doctor might not decrease and, indeed, the presence of the nurse practitioner may stimulate demand to see the doctor. On the other hand, ten hours a week (all that were available to the practices in the Derbyshire study) may not have been enough to satisfy the unmet demand for appointments. Would the results have been the same if a full-time nurse was appointed?

A study on the effect of the introduction of hospital nurse practitioners in helping to reduce junior doctors' hours found little evidence that the doctors *had* reduced their hours. The doctors reported that the intensity of their work rather than actual number of hours worked had declined, and they thought that the quality of services to patients had improved. The authors suggest that effects on junior doctors' workload may increase as the nurse practitioners' confidence and skills improve (Read and Graves, 1994).

Would nurse practitioners be as ineffectual in terms of changing doctors' workloads in general practice as in the hospital setting? It may be equally difficult in the general practice setting to identify, implement and measure the redistribution of workload from doctors to nurse practitioners. There are, however, other precedents. In the case of midwifery, much of the routine antenatal care in many practices has now transferred from the GP to the midwife, and much of the chronic disease management has transferred from the GP to the practice nurse. The answer might lie in a longitudinal study comparing clinical activity between doctors and nurse practitioners. The hypothesis that waits for a doctor's appointment are not affected by the presence of a nurse practitioner could be further tested in situations where the mean wait for an appointment is more than 48 hours, since it has only been tested in this study in situations where the mean wait was less than 48 hours.

Did the presence of an additional nurse practitioner service affect patient satisfaction with the doctor? Patients were asked about their doctor's abilities to listen, explain and provide information, and whether they had enough time with them. Dissatisfaction scores for each of the practices were developed from the data. Three practices improved on their dissatisfaction scores in the second round, two of which were control practices and the other a participating one. The orginal null hypothesis that the nurse practitioner consultation service does not improve the quality of the patient consultation *with the doctor* was therefore not overturned.

The underlying proposition around which the research design was built was that the introduction of another health professional offering additional surgery appointments would ease the burden on the doctors and allow them to concentrate on the clinically more complex cases which were more appropriate for their training and would more closely suit their style of consulting. This would improve patient satisfaction with the consultation. The patient survey results, however, do not show that this was the case, since the overall level of patient satisfaction in the experimental practices did not improve in comparison with the control practices.

Does this mean that the potential for doctors to improve on their patient satisfaction rating is limited? It certainly suggests that, by itself, adding the nurse practitioner to the pool of surgery consultation labour will not result in either improved access to appointments (they will still all be filled) or improved patient satisfaction with consultations provided by doctors. There may be room for improvement if there is a more conscious redistribution of workload and reallocation of time, coupled with further training for doctors in those aspects of the consultation which patients are least happy about. Doctors would also need training in helping them to actively choose their clinical caseload and to help patients to choose to see the nurse practitioner when it is likely that this is more appropriate for them.

One further point on this issue concerns the time that the nurse practitioner was available. The nurse practitioners were able to offer 10 additional hours of consulting time in each of the participating practices (which comprised three, four and five partners). Would the results have been different if the nurses had been full time, offering 30 or so additional consulting hours? It is possible that the redistribution of work, with the doctors assuming a greater proportion of the clinically challenging cases, would then begin to take place, with the potential for improved patient satisfaction.

Time management for doctors

There is evidence from the focus groups with the primary health care teams in the Derbyshire practices that the doctors themselves did not feel that they had more time after the nurse practitioners were introduced. In terms of workload distribution, the doctors in the Ongar Practice felt that they were not doing anything very different from before, but that the nurse practitioner was enabling more patients to be seen: 'It's a resource that would not have been here otherwise and what the [nurse practitioner] sees ... if she hadn't been here, would have had to be seen by us...'. In the Johns Practice the doctors also did not feel that they had any extra time, but although their list size had hardly increased, they seemed to be busier than ever. They put this down to the fact that they were doing more for patients than they had in the past. They mused as to whether, as well as doing more, they were doing more good, but did not reach a conclusion. However, they did feel that they were still enjoying what they were doing. Only in the Sanders Practice, where the nurse practitioner operated a service at the branch surgery, was any difference in workload felt. The doctors thought that they were far less busy at the branch than before the nurse practitioner started, and they noticed a change in what they were doing: the woman doctor used to see only patients with gynaecological problems, and she was now seeing other things, which was a big improvement for her. One of the other doctors estimated that he was seeing fewer children and minor acute illness than before.

Doctors discussed many times their lack of control of their time. They did not have enough time with patients and colleagues, for meetings or for research. One of the doctors highlighted the paradox of ready availability to patients but also the need to adhere to the fixed time of meetings. These were the owners and directors of their enterprise, but they were finding that role difficult to reconcile with being first-point-of-contact practitioners. Allocating additional nurse practitioner appointments did not turn out to provide an opportunity for them to take on something new or to deliver higher quality care. This was probably because the doctors in the focus groups revealed little sense of strategic direction and therefore no clear understanding of how the nurse practitioner might fit into (or not) their vision of the future for primary care. It is interesting to note what things doctors felt they did not have enough time for:

- patients, which patients also feel strongly about

- colleagues

- meetings, which makes for difficulties in team working

- research, which is a recent addition to the GP's repertoire.

Riley notes from her work at the King's Fund with hospital medical directors that they also felt helpless in the face of overwhelming and competing demands on their time. As with GP principals, these are not junior employees but the senior clinicians and respected figures in their organizations with a place on the board (Riley, 1998). Riley suggests that medical training may in itself encourage overcommitment, difficulties in prioritizing and a reluctance to say 'no', characteristics which may be more appropriate to clinical-type tasks rather than management-type tasks.

What did emerge from the focus groups was a growing acknowledgement by the doctors of the role of nurses, not as their assistants, but as complementary providers of care. They recognized that there was a great deal of overlap in the care that could be given as well by nurses as by doctors; and that there was a need to acknowledge and utilize the special skills that each member of the clinical primary health care team had, irrespective of whether they were doctors, nurses or nurse practitioners. The nurses themselves were keen to take on more responsibility, and those in the research who did, felt rewarded. All this looks like a cultural shift away from a masculine and hierarchical model towards a 'flatter' model. But if you flatten completely, how do you coordinate? Following this horizontal logic to its conclusion suggests that primary health care might be ripe for re-engineering. Following Hammer and Champy's definition of this term, which focuses on fundamental rethinking and radical redesign of business processes, in the primary health care context this would comprise both an examination of skill-mix and of the processes in the delivery of primary health care services, and may include nurse partners joining their medical colleagues in a more balanced approach to primary health care management (Hammer and Champy, 1993).

Given that patients have signalled in the research that the style of the nurse practitioner consultation was more acceptable than their doctor's and that they rated her overall care more highly than their doctor's, and that nurses and doctors – with some limits – see the role as an opportunity rather than a threat, is it time that doctors let go a little more of this 'first-point-of-contact' care, as they have in health promotion (to practice nurses) and in maternity care (to midwives) in order to step back and see where primary care is going and to regain some control over their enterprises and their lives? A potential loss may be the personal patient–doctor relationship, but it is under threat anyway. A clarification of priorities may in fact salvage this relationship, particularly for patients at times in their lives when they most need it and would derive most benefit from it. It has been suggested that the patient–doctor relationship may be replaced by the patient–surgery attachment in the way that local people have a loyalty to their local hospital, rather than to a particular clinician or nurse within it (Huntington, 1995). Balint and colleagues argue, from a psychoanalytic perspective, that the close doctor–patient relationship is a mirage: '....we still live in the grip of the myth that general practitioners know their patients well. In reality we only know what patients want us to know. This is quite appropriate... Our knowledge of the patient may range widely, but still remain shallow, until such time that there is a need for a closer doctor–patient relationship, perhaps associated with a crisis for the patient' (Balint *et al.*, 1993). A potential gain for patients in doctors letting go might be the development of the patient–nurse relationship as an alternative, and an enrichment of the quality of primary health care. In a discussion about doctor–patient relationships, Miles discusses the clash between two kinds of expertise: on the one hand there is the professional expertise, based on general rules and categories, learnt during training; and on the other hand there is lay expertise, built from personal experience and that of the social group (Miles, 1991). Nurses, if allowed, may be able to bridge the gap between these sets of expertise by offering to patients an understanding and insight developed from their advocacy role, as well as offering professional care from their clinical skills repertoire.

Significance of GP receptionists

The patient surveys in the Derbyshire Nurse Practitioner Project included an open question, allowing respondents the opportunity to write in a comment of their own choosing. The results from the 'any other comment' question are presented in Figure 4.1 with frequencies relating to the different themes also given. Out of 926 returned questionnaires in the first round of surveys, 289 added some comments (31%). In the second

Figure 4.1   Derbyshire Nurse Practitioner Project: subject frequency of 'any other comments'.

Nature of the consultation (including relationship with doctor)	167
Access to the doctor (including waits for appointment, waits at the surgery and home visiting arrangements)	118
Receptionists	67
Clinical care by doctor	58
Nursing staff (including midwives and health visitors)	32
Practice organization	14
General uncategorized comments (e.g. 'good service', 'better than my last practice')	98

round, out of 886 returned questionnaires, 294 made some comments (33%). There was therefore a total of 583 comments to examine.

The two most frequently mentioned subjects were: first, the nature of the relationship with the doctor particularly in the context of the medical consultation, and second, questions of access to the doctor. This chimes with other patient survey research which indicated that these two areas were of high priority to patients. Perhaps surprisingly, in order of frequency of mention, the third issue that patients felt it was important to mention was receptionists. There were many references to receptionists and also a number relating to 'staff', which in context appeared also to refer to receptionists, for example:

> The pleasant general atmosphere is certainly enhanced by there being a polite, friendly and helpful back-up staff.

There were more favourable than critical comments. Respondents particularly appreciated the helpfulness of receptionists: '[she] ... always has an ear for you'. Also mentioned was their care and compassion, good telephone manner, kindness, friendliness, politeness, consideration, pleasantness and efficiency. Respondents did not like it when receptionists were unhelpful, rude, abrupt, nasty, off-hand or more interested in gossiping with each other. Conversely, there were also adverse comments on the occasions when receptionists appeared to be nosey, overfamiliar and 'tried to be doctors'. There was criticism of the way in which they treated mothers with sick children.

The most interesting point about the receptionist issue in the context of this book is that they still occupy a higher profile as members of the primary health care team than nurses. The role of the receptionist was not discussed in the focus groups with the primary health care teams except insofar as their understanding and acceptance of the nurse practitioner's contribution had an impact on how many patients were booked to see her, and how the availability of additional appointment slots had eased the pressure for the receptionists when trying to meet patient demand. The high profile of receptionists from this survey does suggest that investment in research and development of this role may have a higher than expected impact on patients' views of the quality of primary health care services. If the receptionist role is so crucial, one way forward might be nurses as first-point-of-contact nurse receptionists. This concept is already beginning to be developed in some out-of-hours services, where nurses take the initial call from patients requesting advice or a home visit, and has also been picked up by government in its NHS Direct, the pilot 24-hour advice line to be staffed by nurses.

General practitioners, not general managers

In all three study practices in the Derbyshire Nurse Practitioner Project there was considerable pride in the quality and range of services to patients which they felt they provided, through having high standards and through sheer hard work. One practice aimed to offer appointments for all who requested them within 24 hours, although not necessarily with the doctor of the patient's choice. All mentioned the growth in the health promotion and chronic disease management services as a recent improvement. All three surgeries were modern, well equipped and purpose built and the teams felt that this kind of environment was of help to them and also to their patients. The three practices were therefore positive and confident about the quality of their work before the nurse practitioner was introduced.

The doctors talked at length in the focus groups about what it felt like to work in general practice. They enjoyed the intellectual challenge, although this was admittedly a very small part of the job. They derived personal satisfaction from 'making people better'. They liked the variety in their work. They also enjoyed the element of continuity in general practice, the long-term relationships with patients, their families and the local communities. Less frequently cited but also mentioned was working with a good team. It was clear that the provision of personal clinical care was a source of considerable job satisfaction for the doctors, not only for intellectual reasons, but because they very much enjoyed the constant contact with people. To practise the art of healing and to play a positive and significant part in the lives of their patients was also important to them. They enjoyed their relationship of power and influence which they had with their patients.

On the other hand, the stresses of the job appeared to be growing. They did not like the constant time pressures and in particular, the tension caused, on the one hand, by needing to be constantly accessible to patients, to get through a full surgery, lists of visits and the on-call responsibilities, and on the other hand, also needing to manage the service, including the extra responsibilities of fundholding, working more closely with social services, and the management and development of an ever-increasing complement of staff. There was a need to set priorities and manage time more efficiently. In the Ongar Practice this area was acknowledged as one of the practice's main shortcomings. In the Sanders Practice the senior partner talked about 'too much work', with ever-increasing surgeries, forms to fill in, people on the phone all the time and people 'always wanting you'. In the Johns Practice the following points were made by the doctors, all of whom joined in this discussion:

Researcher: What do you feel you spend too much time on?
Drs A & B: Meetings.
Researcher: Internal meetings?
Dr B: Internal and external.
Dr C: More and more nowadays.
Dr D: I have changed my view entirely over the past year ... I think that the meetings we have now are valuable and productive ... and I see that as an investment of time...
Dr C: I feel that they are valuable, but it rushes you for the other bits, that is what I mean ... the difficulty with meetings is that they are at set times; so if you've got a surgery, with 10 patients or 40 patients ... and ... a meeting at half past eleven ... you have got to rush those 40 people or be late ... that is where it is impinging on my time ... not the intrinsic worth ... if I could go to meetings when I was ready...
Dr B: This is very interesting in a way, because it means that relationships with other professionals in fact take precedence over our dealings with patients...
Dr C: This is the way it feels to me...
Dr D: I dispute that ... because we are not, in fact, each of us, offering a 24-hour 7-day-a-week service: we have time on duty, and time off duty, and we only go to meetings when one of our colleagues are looking on for us...
Dr B: Not always, no...
Dr C: A meeting like this, for instance ... if I had a big list this morning, and a big lot of visits, I would either not come, or do them later in the day, or rush them...
Dr A: Yes, I think what we are talking about here ... what our biggest problem ... my biggest problem more than any single one aspect of my clinical practice, is reconciling the demands of ready accessibility of the doctor with the certain fixed points in my diary, that I accept have to be at these times because

that is when you get the majority of people together ... and that is a cause of stress to me...

What does that discussion show? First, only one of the doctors (Dr D) did not subscribe to the notion that there was a difficulty in juggling meetings with his job of seeing patients. He was the only one to indicate that he saw any *connection* between the 'task' of attending meetings and the 'task' of treating patients. Second, there was a palpable sense of loss of control. The size of surgeries and the number of visits appeared to vary randomly, and probably in the doctors' eyes, in inverse proportion to the management tasks which they faced on a particular day. Yet these were not staff at the bottom of their organization having excessive demands hurled at them by some ruthless boss, they were the directors of their enterprise. In short, they were finding that being practitioners and, at the same time, managing a practice was a tall order. Of the two areas of activity, the 'hands on' work seemed the more important and the more 'natural'. And on the occasions when the two areas appeared as though they were going to collide, they looked on helplessly, wringing their hands at the impossibility of reconciling the competing demands put on them.

Is there a management development training need here? Or is the very success story of general practice forcing these GPs into roles for which they are not only untrained, but to which they are not by nature inclined? Looking at all three practices, there is one doctor in the Ongar Practice who *is* interested in practice development planning, who sees the advent of the nurse practitioner as an opportunity to move away at least from the treatment of acute minor illness, and there is Dr D in the Johns Practice, who tends to think strategically. In the Sanders Practice, the senior partner likened his role in meeting patients' demands to General Custer's problems on the field : '... you shoot a lot of them down, and there is another wave ... they keep coming all the time...'.

The doctors in these three practices did not present themselves, in the way they described their work and their role, as directors of their organizations, although there may have been at least two putative managing directors. In one case, in the Ongar Practice, this doctor was the senior partner, but in the other, the Johns Practice, the putative managing director was not the senior partner. In general practice, that title is still generally attained through age and length of service, rather than any individual management strengths. Instead, the notion of the 'executive partner' is gaining ground, which allows a younger partner to become the 'managing' partner, at the same time as preserving the status (and often the better pay) of the senior partner. There are implications from these findings for the future division of labour in general practice: simply adding nurse practitioners to the equation will not solve the management and leadership conundrum for GPs.

New roles for general practitioners

The Derbyshire study and many others have shown that nurse practitioners can provide an alternative surgery consultation service which is highly regarded by patients and by colleagues. This lends weight to the argument that it is time for doctors to step back from their all-encompassing generalist role. Is it still appropriate for primary health care today? In the US, Mundinger argues that primary medical care no longer requires the level of training that it once did, that there is a increasing gap between specialist and primary care physicians and that therefore there is a growing overlap between primary care physicians and nurses (Mundinger, 1994). The comparison with the US is limited in the sense that most US medicine is specialized. But from the UK perspective Pratt also suggests a scenario with biomedical generalists working alongside other practitioners in primary care (Pratt, 1995). This may also solve the conundrum of GPs working as practitioners and also as directors of their organization. The time may now have come for greater specialization in general practice, in the same way as consultants specialize in different aspects of their speciality, for example, anaesthetists with a special interest in palliative care and oncologists specializing in breast cancer. Hughes argues that continuing education has allowed GPs to become the present-day general physicians, as their consultant colleagues have become super-specialists (Hughes, 1996). There could also be a case for having GPs who do not want management responsibilities, and the potential conflict in values which goes with them, working as practitioners only, alongside colleagues responsible for fundholding, health needs assessment and personnel management (Pratt, 1995).

There is also considerable concern about work and role overload in general practice:

> The general practitioner in the nineties has a more task-sensitive contract, yet has continuing 24 hour responsibility to a patient list, and a burgeoning network of paramedical, social and lay experts with whom he/she is expected to communicate to provide a network of primary provision: curing, caring, rehabilitating, preventing and health promoting. The past emphasis on the continuing doctor–patient relationship is being displaced by an emphasis on teamwork, teambuilding, consumerism, networking, computer-aided communications, sophisticated purchasing skills and commercial incentives ... is the breadth of skills demanded of the new general practitioner so wide that a crash is inevitable? (Stott, 1994)

If we accept the argument that the current situation is not tenable for much longer, because the pressures facing GPs alluded to at the beginning of this book, and the opportunities afforded by the role of the nurse practitioner described later, point to a need for substantial change to organizational arrangements for the delivery of primary health care, it is worth looking in more detail at some alternatives, beginning with alternative models that unpack the all-encompassing generalist responsibilities which all general practitioners currently have. How could the roles of primary care doctor be divided in the future, and how would these roles fit with the nurse practitioner providing an alternative surgery consultation service? Five roles can be identified:

- biomedical generalist

- clinical specialist

- management specialist

- commissioning specialist

- subprincipal.

These roles are described in more detail below.

Patients place a high value on ease of access to a doctor's appointment when they decide that they need one. Therefore, the first role that is required is that of the *biomedical generalist*, to use Pratt's term (Pratt, 1995). This doctor would principally make use of the scientific method to provide medical care. This relies on applying existing medical knowledge and using probability predictions to arrive at specific decisions during the course of the patient consultation about diagnosis, prognosis and treatment. This kind of consultation is likely to be fairly short, and therefore the nature of the job would allow a high throughput of patients. By offering a high-volume service this job would meet continuing patient pressure for ease of access to doctor appointments. Further, although there has been criticism from patients of the shortness of the doctor consultation, there must surely still be a place for the swift patient–doctor interaction. When, for example, the patient requires a straightforward decision about diagnosis or reassurance about a minor concern, a more comprehensive biographical inquiry, such as developed by Balint (Balint, 1957), or the offer of emotional or spiritual support would be misplaced and may even put patients off.

The kind of GP who suits this role is one who tends to the shorter consultation, likes variety and is relatively fearless of uncertainty and the unknown. They are likely not to mind being on-call too much, because they are able to 'switch off' immediately after the visit or call. They are happy to make a series of fast decisions and they obtain intellectual satisfaction from working on complex issues at speed to a high level of accuracy. What they are less keen on are the longer consultations, especially where the illness is poorly defined, and where social and emotional problems play an important part. There are examples of biomedical generalists in the focus groups conducted as part of the Derbyshire Nurse Practitioner Project.

The strength of the biomedical generalists is that they offer an appropriate first port of call for any medical problem. They think and act speedily, and are able to deal effectively with the high and increasing volume of work in general practice, particularly in the general surgery. Their major weakness is in not being able to adequately provide for the other aspects of the consultation which certainly some patients require, especially the caring, biographical and spiritual aspects (Pratt, 1995). They may be doctors who do not get to know their patients well. Some biomedical generalist work, especially the diagnosis and treatment of minor illness, was successfully taken on by the three nurse pracitition ers in this study and it seems likely, in view of the acceptability of the model above, that nurses will carry out more of this type of work. It remains the case, however, that one of the key strengths of medical education is that it does provide the knowledge base and the training for the utilization of the scientific method in diagnosis and treatment of disease to a level of sophistication which nursing education cannot reach. Therefore for consultations where the medical condition itself is the primary concern, rather than the condition plus the other relating physical, emotional and social factors, the biomedical generalist is likely to be the most appropriate person to go to.

Many doctors indicate that they have already carved out areas of particular expertise, as a way of meeting patient need for high-quality care, and as a way of pursuing personal academic and research interests. Irvine recommends that GPs also develop special clinical interests as a way of delivering more care of high technical quality which will be required in the move from less hospital to more community-based care (Irvine, 1993). The second role would therefore be that of the *clinical specialist* within general practice. This is akin to the hospital specialist who focuses on a particular area within their speciality, as well as treating some patients across the range of conditions falling within their main speciality. Clinical specialization within general practice might be in, for example, child health, maternity, minor surgery, family planning, health problems of the elderly, mental health, chronic and long-term disease surveillance, and so on. As the boundaries of primary care widen, there will be an increasing need for some degree of specialization. In the Derbyshire study with the focus groups it became clear that some of the doctors, especially in the Johns Practice, had already carved out areas of interest and specialization; for example, the doctor who complained about being brought social problems which he could not deal with was also the one who particularly liked and did a lot of minor surgery. In group practices, which are increasingly the norm, this provides patients with the opportunity, but not the necessity, of seeing different doctors according to what is wrong with them. Many doctors say, anecdotally, that patients frequently avail themselves of this choice. The other advantage for patients is that some degree of specialization should lead to higher clinical standards of care, as these clinical specialists develop expertise in particular areas.

The kind of doctor who would be attracted to this role is one who likes going into some depth over a clinical problem and who feels frustrated by the constraints of the standard 5–10 minute consultation. They are likely to handle well the presentation of additional social and emotional complications connected with the medical problem. The advantage for these doctors is the intellectual stimulation provided by acquiring a more in-depth knowledge of a particular clinical area as a counterbalance to the day-to-day generalist work. They may carry out audit or research on behalf of the practice on the subject and interface with the secondary care specialists to clarify joint care or referral protocols. The research with the focus groups demonstrated that practice nurses and nurse practitioners in the study practices were also specializing in certain areas: for example, in HRT, asthma, diabetes, family planning. They particularly enjoyed this aspect of their work, and were considered the 'practice specialists' in these subjects, not the 'nurse specialists'. This suggests that specialist roles in primary care should be considered not merely as an issue for doctors, but also for nurses.

One problem with the role is that overfocus on the area of specialization may lead to a loss of expertise in other areas. This may leave the practice somewhat exposed. For example, a GP who deals with a lot of psychosocial and mental health problems may not see enough acute illness to be able to diagnose and treat safely. An associated difficulty would be the loss of flexibility of cover: if one doctor was the maternity specialist for the practice, and was on holiday at the time of a complication, the practice would be unable – if the example was beyond the capability of the midwife – to help their patient, who would then have to be referred to the secondary level of care.

Some doctors acquire 'speciality labels' without actively seeking out patients with those particular problems. In other words, *patients* decide that a certain doctor is particularly appopriate to deal with a certain set of problems. The woman doctor in the Ongar Practice, who tended to see less acute illness and a greater proportion of patients with psychosocial problems, experienced this. Indeed, this is particularly the case with women doctors who, because many patients prefer to see doctors of their own gender, see a disproportionate amount of women and a high proportion of gynaecological problems. These doctors get pigeonholed and do not always like this. The woman doctor in the Sanders Practice focus groups welcomed the nurse practitioner model because it meant that she was no longer seeing so many patients with women's health problems and was also able to share those whom she did see on an ongoing basis with the nurse practitioner. It emerged that this doctor's area of interest was actually elderly people who were mentally frail.

It is also possible that specialization will lead to lack of continuity of care and loss of the personal and holistic family doctor relationship with patients, which doctors and patients both appear to value. It has, however, already been argued above that, with the expanded primary health care team and the advent of group practice, this continuity of care may already be illusory for all but a minority of patients at a time of their lives when they most need it, for example, with severe, ongoing, degenerative or terminal health problems. Instead, the clinical specialist role within general practice does offer patients the opportunity to consult within primary care a doctor known to them and who has more experience and more advanced and up-to-date knowledge of the condition than one might normally expect. This second role would also fit well with the nurse practitioner model described above. Patients would be able to choose to consult with either the doctor or the nurse practitioner for common illnesses and minor complaints, and choose to see the doctor for particular health problems in which they were known to have developed special interest and expertise. This happens currently in the US where a proportion of family physicians are specialists. The research demonstrated that nurses too were specializing within primary care; patients might choose to see the nurse practitioner over a menopause problem, if she was known to be the practice specialist in that area.

There are problems for doctors not only in their clinical roles, but in their management roles. It became clear in the course of the analysis of the focus groups that doctors experienced considerable tension between the demands created by patients (surgeries, home visits, on-call), the demands created by being responsible for a growing business and the expectations of the wider NHS. Since the research was carried out it now appears that GPs are also supposed to be leaders not only of their own small organizations, but also of the NHS, if one interprets literally the publication of *Towards a Primary Care-led NHS* (NHS Executive, 1994) and subsequent policy documents including *The New NHS* White Paper (NHS Executive, 1997).

Irvine has suggested that management responsibilities should be defined as additional rather than core work for GPs (Irvine, 1993). The third role could therefore be that of the *management specialist* within general practice. The aim would be to have a properly recognized role for these doctors away from the clinical arena, as managers or directors of an aspect of their business. The management specialist posts might be in information technology, personnel management, financial affairs or interagency relations. These are all areas where attention and expertise are required in greater measure than currently available from the full-time clinical doctor. Following doctor training in these roles, the practice would then have a professional management resource to match the clinical expertise and which would be appropriate to the size of the organization; medium-sized practices now have a staff complement of 30 or so inclusive of attached staff. This new role raises the issue of who should lead the new primary health care organization: should it be the executive partner who has developed chairmanship skills in his management specialist role or should it be the practice manager? The answer probably lies in seeking local solutions, depending on the skills within the practice management team. Huntington argues that there are three routes into management for GPs: first, as partners they are directors of the practice even if they wish to concentrate on clinical work; second, they could become GPs with a part-time management portfolio in areas such as staffing or information technology; and third, they could become the managing or executive partner (Huntington, 1995). Even in this last situation, Huntington suggests that a pairing of the management function between the practice manager and the executive partner is the most appropriate arrangement.

The kind of doctor who would be attracted to a management specialist role is one who is getting somewhat tired of routine surgery work and may have already found that they enjoy the organization and management part of their current work as a partner. One such doctor can be found in the Johns Practice focus groups. In contrast to colleagues, he claims to understand the place, purpose and value of having meetings. There are also the doctors who enjoy computing, and many practices now harbour such enthusiasts. Others volunteer to serve in medical representative organizations. The consequences on morale of a lack of a career trajectory for GPs have been pointed out (McBride and Metcalfe, 1995). An explicitly recognized move into management may be a solution to this and to early 'burnout', which Kirwan and Armstrong have uncovered (Kirwan and Armstrong, 1995).

The disadvantage of the development of this role is that doctors would be taken away from what they were trained for. Tudor Hart would argue that GP training has fitted within the 'Osler paradigm' and is too restrictive anyway, that the 'doctor-centred, episodic technical fix' has limited clinical effectiveness and that accountability to the whole community is a core responsibility for GPs (Tudor Hart, 1988). There is a question mark over whether it has to be doctors who carry out practice-based health needs assessment. Some practices employ public health nurses to do this work. Meanwhile, health visitors have received training to do this, but do not often get the opportunity to practise these skills or to disseminate findings and discuss them with the primary health care team.

In any event, doctors would be unlikely to want to be full-time management specialists and may opt for a way of working which is closer to the clinical director model now popular in secondary care. The lessons learnt from the development and early experiences of that model could serve to improve on that prototype for primary health care and build a doctor–manager role in which relations with peers and colleagues are better defined, and where time management between the clinical and directorship roles is clear.

The fourth role for doctors is as *commissioning specialist*. This role could develop from the current pool of expertise among GPs in fundholding, health needs assessment and locality commissioning. In the Ongar Practice the doctor describes leaving the treatment of minor illness behind – to the nurse practitioner – in order to take on new work in health needs assessment. Tudor Hart emphasizes the importance of this new role for GPs, as a way of moving towards the care of whole populations, in addition to providing care to complaining individuals, and using the opportunities provided by having registered populations and practice computers on which to manipulate and extract data (Tudor Hart, 1988). The White Paper *The New NHS* (NHS Executive, 1997) envisages GPs and community nurses working together in primary care groups serving populations of about 100 000 to commission services, and states that GPs who take on key responsibilities within primary care groups will be appropriately reimbursed.

The fifth role for doctors is as the *subprincipal*. This role has already been mooted by NAHAT in its proposals for change to GP vocational training arrangements (NAHAT, 1994), which would bring GP training more closely into line with the model for the training of hospital consultants. The RCGP and NAHAT both suggest that full training (higher professional training) should be increased from three to five years, and that the normal standard for GP principals should be the MRCGP qualification (RCGP, 1994). The first three years (the general professional training) would prepare doctors for posts of 'assistant' or 'associate' in general practice. Some doctors could choose to remain as assistants and not proceed to the principal grade. Irvine also advocates this role for doctors who do not wish to progress in general practice beyond the core responsibilities of basic clinical care and health promotion (Irvine, 1993).

In addition to this two-tier approach to the training of 'career' GPs, other opportunities could be opened up for doctors in training to go into general practice. It should be possible not only for the vocational training scheme registrars, who may only have had two years post-registration hospital training, but also for other more experienced junior doctors to spend time as GPs. This group of doctors may choose later in their career to go into general practice, they may not yet have decided where they will specialize or they may decide that a spell in primary care, with the insights that it may offer, would enhance their knowledge, skills and understanding of the hospital speciality that they have already chosen to follow. Specialities which may benefit from a better understanding of the primary care perspective include obstetrics, care of the elderly and mental health, where so much care is carried out within the primary setting. Increasingly, however, as the boundaries are pulled back, for example, with the increase in the management of chronic disease away from the hospital setting and the spread of the hospital-at-home schemes, it may be advantageous for doctors in training in general medicine and general surgery to spend time in general practice. After all, GP trainees spend time as junior doctors in various hospital specialities. It makes sense that if this training is relevant to them, work in primary medical care would be relevant for the future consultants of these same specialities.

This role, which would be similar in grading and seniority to the hospital registrar or senior registrar, would promote closer relations between the primary and secondary levels, since these doctors would often have inside knowledge of the local hospitals and may subsequently return to work there. A similar case could be made for doctors in training to become public health consultants spending time in general practice as subprincipals. The practices would benefit from public health expertise and knowledge of the role of commissioning groups and of health authorities. The future public health consultants would go back to work in their local health authorities with insight about general practice and the local population's health needs, as well as with positive relationships developed with some local GPs who, in line with a primary-care led NHS, will increasingly – in theory at least – be working in primary care groups to identify and meet local health priorities. It also makes sense for doctors training to be GPs to work as public health doctors as part of their training, to equip them to carry out practice-based needs asssessments.

The quality of clinical care within general practice would improve because some of the subprincipals would bring with them an advanced clinical understanding of the speciality which they came from. This could benefit patients in two ways, both because the care given by the subprincipals (for some conditions) would be expert and because the partners could learn from the additional clinical expertise of these colleagues. The role might also produce cost savings as a subprincipal grade would be paid less than a partner. These doctors may also be at a stage in their career and personal lives where the burden of the night on-call appears to them less onerous than it does to their GP colleagues.

One disadvantage of the role is the potential risk the practice might be taking in letting a doctor not trained in general practice work without supervision. It is in the nature of general practice for much clinical work to be undertaken in isolation from colleagues, a point made by one of the doctors in the Sanders Practice. The other doctors may have difficulty in trusting them, just as in the same practice the doctors demurred at the idea of an unknown nurse, even with appropriate diplomas, doing the kind of nurse practitioner work which they had entrusted to their erstwhile practice nurse. An additional disadvantage might be a perceived lack of loyalty to the organization if the job was considered a stepping stone or if it was structured in such a way that, as with the very junior hospital doctor posts, there was no long-term post available or job security of any kind.

There is a risk too that there may be role overlap or conflict with other members of the primary health care team; for example, one subprincipal who was a former obstetrics registrar might clash with the practice midwife or another who was a psychiatric registrar might clash with the practice counsellor. There is no evidence, however, that vocational training scheme trainees have this difficulty, and the role may in fact have the opposite effect, with the various non-medical clinical specialists within the team using the presence of a doctor with some special knowledge of their area to their own and their patients' advantage. The nurse practitioner model which has been explored in this book would work with the subprincipal role, as both could run surgery consultation services, but there may be greater areas of role overlap; for example, patients may see both as an alternative to bothering the (principal) doctor.

This argument leads to the risk that patients would identify two classes of GP and choose to see the principal rather than the assistant, in the same way that they prefer to see the hospital consultant rather than their registrar. To obviate this potential for hierarchical classification, the subprincipal role would have to be promoted positively. A precedent within general practice has, however, already been set with the introduction of the nurse practitioner role, which the primary health care teams themselves identified not as offering patients a doctor substitute, but as offering something different – a health practitioner with particular interests, skills and areas of specialization – and therefore offering patients an enhanced choice. The patients' survey results from various studies suggest that this role interpretation and promotion has worked as far as patients are concerned.

In addition to this study of different GP roles within primary medical care, it is worth considering the different organizational structures within which they might fit. GP principals in the current arrangement are all partners in a business; an option for the future might be for some doctors to be salaried and employed by the partnership, which would suit doctors who would prefer not to enter either the financial or managerial responsibilities of a partnership, or to have salaried doctors employed by a health authority that itself acts in place of the partnership of a practice. A further option is the polyclinic model of care with doctors, salaried or self-employed, working alongside other health professionals in a reinvention of the health centre approach. Polyclinics can offer, in isolation or in combination, primary health care, consultant outpatient clinics, day surgery, minor casualty or multisectoral services.

One example of a polyclinic in the UK is the South Westminster Centre for Health (Gordon and Hadley, 1996), where the particular variant of the polyclinic model includes the provision of general practice services, consultant clinics and a nurse practitioner minor treatment service. Another variant would be nurse or medical registrar triage to ensure that patients with the most clinically complex cases received appropriate and effective medical attention. A further possibility is a fundamental redesign of the primary care service by looking at patients' preferences and clinically effective treatments, re-examining care pathways, selecting the most appropriate care package and then identifying the most appropriate professional to undertake it. This has been undertaken partially in a study of users' views of antenatal maternity services in the community. It was found that the first point of contact within the NHS for a pregnant woman was her doctor, but that in view of who she considered was in charge of her care (the midwife) and the importance to the woman of that first consultation confirming the pregnancy, it should be the midwife not the doctor who was offered as a first point of contact (Chambers, 1995b). Initial responses to this recommendation have been lukewarm even from midwives, suggesting that displacing the family doctor as a first point of contact and introducing triage would not yet be acceptable in primary care.

These roles are offered as alternatives to the all-encompassing and overburdening role with which GPs are currently struggling, with the prospect of still more responsibility as key agents in the primary care-led NHS being heaped upon them. The proposal for these roles is drawn from a number of sources. First, there are the difficulties which GPs find themselves in. Second, there is the new opportunity for sharing work in a different way with nurse practitioners, which has been identified as a way forward, particularly in circumstances where there is either a high list size, high consulting rates, a branch surgery, a single-handed practice or no woman partner. Third, there are the recommendations for changes in undergraduate and postgraduate medical training, for example the GMC's *Tomorrow's Doctors* (GMC, 1993) and the RCGP's *Education and Training for General Practitioners* (RCGP, 1994), which have a bearing on the kind of hospital and community doctors envisaged in the future. Finally, there is the analysis provided from within the GP profession about the need for change, for example, Tudor Hart's perspective on the limits of the 'Osler paradigm' (Tudor Hart, 1988) and Irvine's view of future developments in general practice (Irvine, 1993). The RCGP too has acknowledged the value of some specialization in clinical or management areas, as long as all GPs continue to have high levels of competence in areas of high usage or high risk and adequate competence across the full range (RCGP, 1996).

The underlying principle is that, for the benefit of patients, these roles should play to individual doctors' strengths. Some doctors are keen to meet the challenges of commissioning, computing or some degree of clinical specialization. Others are not. Some doctors complain of the trivia of general surgery, but others would prefer not to be taken away from this day-to-day work to spend time in lengthy meetings about practice strategy, commissioning or arrangements for collaboration which they struggle to understand. Some doctors have difficulty in dealing with social and emotional problems brought by their patients, others recognize this as one of their strengths. It is time to recognize that no single individual can excel at the whole range of activities now required within general practice, and it is therefore sensible to share the work out according to preferences and strengths. Effective teamwork in primary health care, for which role clarification is a prerequisite, has been emphasized for some time and continues to receive attention (for example, DHSS, 1971; Pritchard and Pritchard, 1994; Pendleton, 1995). The exact distribution of roles would vary from practice to practice according to size, personalities and organization needs. For example, one doctor may be the commissioning lead and the practice clinical specialist in maternity, as well as taking part in running some general surgeries. He is unlikely to see large numbers of patients in a surgery, however, in the way a biomedical generalist would. These roles would complement the development of a nurse practitioner role, building from practice-based patient needs and professional strengths.

New primary care organizations

What new model of primary health care provision emerges from these role developments? Orchestrated by the WHO, a world vision for primary health care was created with the Alma Ata declaration in 1977 and was reinforced by *Health For All by the Year 2000* targets. At a national level this was belatedly followed by the publication of the *Health of the Nation* policy document, although this provided targets rather than structures and means (Department of Health, 1992). There is now also a government vision for a primary care-led NHS (NHS Executive, 1994, 1997), however hazy and still very much 'work-in-progress', but there is not yet, within the overall developing scheme of things, a clearly defined vision for the organization of primary care itself. This could be contrasted with conceptualizations of the hospitals of the future, where there has been discussion about role, size and features. In a number of local initiatives, for example in Cheshire (Chambers, 1996a), GPs are being encouraged to think strategically and to plan the future direction for their enterprise. But as well as training and support, they need a framework within which they can sensibly operate and on which they can pin their strategy.

Some of the key findings in this book are:

- nurse practitioners can provide first-point-of-contact primary health care which is acceptable to their professional colleagues and highly acceptable to patients; in particular nurse practitioners offer the possibility of a more relaxed and less hurried consultation which patients value

- the presence of nurse practitioners may have some impact on the nature of the work of doctors, more probably so as the ratio of nurse practitioner to doctor approaches 1:1

- the presence of nurse practitioners does not in itself improve the quality of the medical consultation from the patients' perspective or improve patients' assessments of the overall care given by their doctor; other measures will be necessary to address patient-perceived deficiencies in the medical consultation

- GPs may be struggling in their role as directors of their enterprise, and in their role as deliverers of a biopsychosocial model of primary care; alternative roles for GPs have been suggested in a new study, to complement the new role emerging for nurses.

These findings suggest that a number of organizational changes in the supporting infrastructure of primary care are required. Developing out of the present practices, primary health care teams and learning from the research findings, primary care organizations (PCOs) would be the setting and focal point for the provision of primary care. Care would be provided on a multidisciplinary basis, operating on the principle that the most appropriate professional should take the lead worker role, according to patient choice, professional training and organizational demands. Nurse practitioners would be lead workers in the monitoring of chronic illness and for much first-point-of-contact work. GPs would continue to be directly accessible to patients, but would focus on, and be chosen by, patients needing help with the more serious acute, intractable or long-term conditions. Hospital services would be seen as supporting primary care in the spirit of the Alma Ata declaration (WHO, 1978), rather than being on a higher plane, and dealing with the residual health care problems not containable by promotion, prevention or treatment within the primary care setting. Local health authorities would regulate and support PCOs. In view of the tremendous power, influence, control and resources invested in PCOs, these authorities would have commensurately powerful tools for monitoring the quality of services they provide. Contracts would no longer be placed with individual GPs but with the PCOs, following recommendations made by the new local commissioning bodies, the primary care groups, as envisaged in the White Paper *The New NHS* (NHS Executive, 1997).

What would it feel like for patients registered with PCOs? They would see doctors for their health problems less often, for example, not for pregnancy or long-term chronic conditions, but when they did, the consultations would be longer. Older and iller people, in particular, would have better access to doctors than they do now. Patients would have a better understanding of the range of skills which nurses have. They would not be likely to say to a family member or neighbour, 'Have you been to the doctor's yet for that rash/cough/worry/checkup?', but rather, 'Have you checked that out at the PCO?'.

What would it be like to be GPs in a PCO? It is likely that they would feel more in control of their lives, although paradoxically they would have relinquished power to nursing colleagues and to the PCO management board. There would be a number of reasons for this feeling of greater control: first, the workload would be more sensibly and reasonably divided; second, monitoring by external agencies, principally the local health authority, would be overt rather than covert; and third, they and the PCO would be clearer about the direction in which they were heading, because each PCO would work to a development plan agreed with the primary care group and the health authority. The tension created by having a personal contract with the health authority but accountability to a partnership and a practice population, as described by Irvine, would have disappeared (Irvine, 1993). GPs would aim to offer patients longer consultations, including a discussion, where applicable, of referral arrangements, rather than merely an explanation of the decision. GPs would still aim to stay on a long-term basis in their PCO as they did when in a practice partnership, so that they would still be able to offer continuity of care to families along with their nursing colleagues. They would be supported by subprincipals who would be less likely to fill permanent posts in PCOs.

Nurses would discover that they were able to push back the boundaries of the limits to their care, and would routinely examine, diagnose, prescribe and treat as part of their remit. They would find that patients and professional colleagues have a much better understanding of their role and acceptance of their expanded responsibilities. They would also have places on the PCO management board, as equity partners and salaried partners, to reflect their enhanced contribution. The whole nursing team, including midwives, health visitors and district nurses, would be direct employees or partners of the PCO.

How would such an organization, with up to 40 staff, be managed? First, there would be a board, consisting of equity and salaried medical and nursing partners and an elected patient representative. The board would be chaired by the executive partner and led by the chief executive (the erstwhile practice manager role). The board would be responsible for four broad areas:

- strategy and monitoring, producing the PCO development plans and annual reports

- research into clinical effectiveness, patient satisfaction and efficiency

- health needs assessment

- interagency relations including representation on the local primary care group.

Members of the board would be the management specialists referred to above, from nursing, medical and other disciplines. They would be directors of specific aspects of the organization, for example, health needs assessment, research, operations, staffing and HR, and finance. The remainder of the medical staff (including biomedical generalists and subprincipals) would be accountable to one of the directors on the board. There would be no 'middle management'. Staff would be encouraged to work across a number of directorates to avoid the scourge of interdepartmental rivalries and hostilities.

Such an organization might be better suited to the challenges, pressures and opportunities of primary care in circumstances in which the health service itself, its public and their government all see primary care as the cornerstone. The question posed at the start of this book was whether it was appropriate for GPs to continue to act as the first point of contact for patients seeking help with a health problem and as the gatekeepers to secondary services. The book set out to explore and evaluate an alternative model, involving a new nurse role – the nurse practitioner – in which patients could choose to see either the GP or the nurse. The findings suggest that this alternative model is viable. But the findings also suggest that there are other unresolved quality and organizational issues for primary care. The PCO proposed above addresses these issues and incorporates a much more high-profile role for nurses, including not only the role as alternative first point of contact for patients, but also the authority to refer to secondary care and board level management responsibility. What is needed now is an evaluation of this new organization, focusing on its acceptability to patients and to the professionals.

5 The nurse practitioner role: professional implications for doctors and nurses

Training

In all three practices in the Derbyshire Project, the nurse practitioners explained how they had sat in on doctors' surgeries. In the Ongar Practice, they had concentrated on the morning surgeries, which contained the type of health problems that it was anticipated the nurse practitioner was going to be facing, that is, minor acute illness. In the Sanders Practice, the nurse sat in with all the partners in turn. She was so enthusiastic about the experience that the practice nurses approached the doctors to ask if they too could do this.

In the Johns and Sanders Practices they had developed detailed protocols. Part of the reason for this, particularly in the Sanders Practice, was to address the medico-legal issues, because the practice felt that it could not demonstrate in any other way what standards the nurse was working to in the absence of an externally recognized course. The problem was that they could not develop a sufficient number of protocols to encompass the wide variety of work that the nurse was doing.

In the Ongar Practice the nurse practitioner felt that there was a lack of relevant external training courses to meet her needs. By the second group discussion she thought that the lack of training was the principal hindrance to the development of her role, and this included both internally organized training opportunities, such as tutorials on certain topics, externally organized sessions and a formal academic course.

In the Johns Practice training did not emerge as an issue during the group discussions. But in the Sanders Practice the main problem was the investment of time. As well as sitting in on surgery consultations, the development of protocols had necessitated one-to-one tutorials with the doctor mentor. These had been fruitful. This practice reported at the second group discussion how they had used the idea of the tutorial system for training the practice nurses in their extended roles of managing chronic disease, and it had been a success. But the doctor mentor was doubtful whether they had the organizational capacity to train a nurse practitioner all over again:

> I don't know whether we would do what we have done, again ... there is too much work involved ... I have enjoyed doing it ... I have learnt a lot from doing it, but a tremendous amount of time has gone into it ... I would be a mentor again, if there was some other course ... but all the tutorials ... the anatomy, and treatment ... it took a lot of time ... I wouldn't do it again ... I've got too much to do...

The other concern was about the lack of a paper and therefore a portable qualification. In the Sanders Practice, they described how at the nurse practitioner conference in Colorado, USA, which the three Derbyshire nurses attended one year, they felt keenly that they could not prove what standards the nurses had reached, whereas all the other participants, including the other group from the UK, had or were studying for a recognized qualification. Other partners in the Sanders Practice made the point that the diploma would not necessarily mean that the nurse would be, practically speaking, proficient. From their point of view, the fact that the nurse had been trained by one of their colleagues gave them more confidence than a diploma. They agreed that a combination of practical experience, something like a vocational training scheme with an assessment by the partners, and a diploma would be the most comprehensive form of training.

This question of not knowing how their colleagues, including the nurse practitioner, in the primary health care team performed because of the privacy of the consultation vexed one of the partners in the Sanders Practice:

> ...one of the things about us as GPs is that we think we know how our partners practise ... but in actual fact we sit in our rooms and work in very solitary situations ... we have their written comments, we have a feel for the way they handle things, but in fact we know very little ... to some extent, that also goes for the way our practice nurses, the way our nurse practitioner works, we can only judge things by what is left, by the results and by patients' attitudes ... and to some extent patient questionnaires would form a valid way of assessing whether patients' perceived needs had been met...

Training for the nurse practitioner was a problem in the Derbyshire Project because of the time investment for the practices; there were no tailor-made nurse practitioner courses available at that time locally or nationally. There was a further concern that external training courses for nurse practitioners, while conferring a recognized and portable qualification, would not be sufficient to engender trust in the doctors employing a nurse practitioner. What are doctors looking for in their new nursing colleagues? They want to be convinced that these are professionals who will not let them or themselves down. This calls for assertiveness and inner confidence from reflective and constructively critical practitioners. The nurse practitioner role also calls for strong communication, management and interpersonal skills in addition to the extra technical skills required for safe examination, diagnosis and treatment of minor illness. This is a tall order and a barrier to the further development of this role. The time investment for practices to carry out their own training where the nurses do not have access to a taught course is considerable. On the other hand, the evidence points to doctors wanting a large say in the training. One solution, mooted by Martin, suggests that faculties of the RCGP might mount courses in conjunction with the RCN; a more local solution might be clusters of practices organized to share the training burden, with the support of local trusts and commissioning authorities (Martin, 1991). Another solution appears to be a combination of the externally provided and validated course, such as the one now franchised by the RCN, with practice-based training with a GP mentor in order for the nurse's colleagues to develop confidence in sharing clinical decision making with a non-medical colleague.

The Scope of Professional Practice issued by the nurses' national training and regulatory body, the UKCC, in 1992 addresses the issue of training more fundamentally: it removes the inhibitor which had been that any extension of role required official 'certification' (PL/CNO(89)10). The UKCC argument is based on the notion that piecemeal training courses and certificates of competence detract from the importance of holistic care and prevent nurses from fulfilling their potential for the benefit of patients (UKCC, 1994). This opens a way forward for nurses to develop and expand their professional practice and their role without necessarily going on courses. It remains to be seen how easily the culture shift will be achieved; nurses are used to the comfort and security of feeling appropriately trained precisely because they have completed a particular course. This study also demonstrated that some doctors feel uneasy about nurses practising in areas of expertise for which they have not received certificated training. What is the answer?

The UKCC has suggested a framework for continuing professional development of nurses which would fit with the nurse practitioner model of primary care (UKCC, 1993). They suggest three levels of nurses: registered, specialist and advanced. The nurse practitioner offering an alternative surgery consultation service would need to be at the specialist or advanced level. There is no reason to suppose that some of her nursing colleagues on the primary health care team would not be functioning at this level as well; this would also go some way to assuage concerns about a supernurse elite. Without returning to the pre-*Scope of Professional Practice* era, reassurance for medical colleagues that the nurses were able to work safely at this level would need to be given, possibly in the form of a credit accumulation system, and the nurses themselves would need a system of recognized advanced qualifications to demonstrate their level of competence to prospective employers.

Nurse practitioner courses are now being introduced all over the UK. By 1997 there were some 300 qualified nurse practitioners in the UK, and a similar number currently in educational programmes leading to the nurse practitioner qualification (Johnson, 1997). The training conundrum would appear to be solved, but there is a fly in the ointment: seven years after the RCN established the first training course for nurse practitioners, the UKCC has not yet recognized the title or role. This means that the term 'nurse practitioner' is not a recognized nursing role at either specialist or advanced practitioner level. As Campbell argues, in doing this, the UKCC risk the criticism that they have failed to meet their duty to protect the public by ensuring that all nurse practitioners are appropriately educated and experienced to take on such a role (Campbell, 1997). In addition, nurse practitioners may be denied prescribing rights (unless they qualify on other grounds) and yet if they hold the RCN degree they will have studied pharmacology to a higher level than those currently able to prescribe under the pilot schemes.

The failure of the UKCC to recognize the nurse practitioner title is no mere oversight, nor can it be ascribed to the fact that the term 'nurse practitioner' itself is woolly, ambiguous and misleading; it probably is – but no one has yet thought of a better one. The UKCC's approach is no less than a reflection of many nurses' and doctors' own sense of ambiguity about a job which looks increasingly like a potent medley of their very separate professions. It is possible that the introduction of this 'alternative consultant' could destabilize roles and relations between these two groups, which have carved out distinctive roles and survived cohabitation, albeit unequally and sometimes uneasily, for many decades on the hospital ward and more recently in the doctor's surgery. What is the evidence to support this argument?

Status problems

The focus groups conducted during the Derbyshire Nurse Practitioner Project provide some useful material around changing relationships between doctors and nurses in primary care. The first point to be made is that the process of defining a clear and distinct role was an important issue for each professional group in the team. Although they were not specifically asked to, the doctors and nurses in each group discussion spent time on this before they felt able to move on to debating the impact of the nurse practitioner.

The nurse practitioners and the doctors described their changing professional relationships. In the Johns Practice, the doctor mentor remarked that they spent a lot more time talking about things that they would not have talked about before. For the nurse in the Sanders Practice it was an eye-opener, during the training period, to be able to sit in on the doctor–patient consultation, which she had never before done as a nurse. Two aspects of the consultation struck her especially forcefully: first, the amount of trivial things that patients brought to the doctor, and second, the speed at which the doctors worked. The doctors also described the effect it had on them, as a non-training practice, of having someone sit in on the consultations:

> ...It has been very interesting having her sit in, because it makes you think about what you are doing. And it makes you justify it a bit more. You don't cut as many corners...

Another doctor explained how nice it felt having another professional in the same room to bounce ideas off after consulting in isolation for six years. The discussion then turned to the thought that the nurse practitioner could do some of the things which the doctors did, and would the government move towards the substitution of doctors with nurse practitioners because they were cheaper. The conversation continued like this:

NP: So you see me as a threat...
GP1: Well, no...
GP2: You won't be a threat to me, but you may be a threat to other GPs in the future...
GP3: At the end of the day, we are very expensive...
GP1: We are...
GP3: We are expensive to train, and expensive in what we do...
GP2: We are very well trained though...
GP1: We are probably overtrained for what we do...
GP2: So therefore, three of them for one of us ... they are going to look at that....

In the Ongar Practice the nurse mentioned that, over time, her relationship with the doctors had changed slightly, generally becoming more relaxed and trusting. One of the doctors had double-checked all her work rigorously before signing any prescription in the first few weeks, but he was now saying things like: 'You know more about this than I do' or 'You are getting good at this'.

In terms of workload distribution, the doctors in the Ongar Practice felt that they were not doing anything very different from before, but that the nurse practitioner was enabling more patients to be seen. In the Johns Practice the doctors also did not feel that they had any extra time, but although their list size had hardly increased, they seemed to be busier than ever. In the Sanders Practice the doctors thought that they were far less busy at the branch than before the nurse practitioner started.

As well as talking about changing relationships between the doctors and the nurse practitioner, each practice also talked about changes in relations between doctors and nurses generally in primary care, and the prospects for a more widespread extension of nursing roles. In the Johns Practice one of the doctors said that he would like to see the nurse practitioner experiment extended to other practice nurses, if they wanted it. The senior partner in the same practice described how professional relationships between the doctors and nurses were changing, particularly in the way in which doctors referred patients to nurses:

> ...one is less and less asking nurses to do so-and-so specifically ... you say 'There is a problem, get on with it', ... things that seem appropriate ... and they seem happy to take their own decisions on that...

In the same practice the doctor mentor talked about the shifts over time in thinking and in the dynamics of the primary health care team:

> I think this is a continuum from the days of the 1965 Charter ... before that time doctors did everything, and the nurses were designed to help and to do things for the doctor ... gradually with the expansion of teams, what has happened here, particularly in the last couple or three years, is that we have recognized each other's abilities more, and each other's limitations, and the tasks that are carried out nowadays are much more related to the skills and abilities of the person carrying them out. I think sensitivities have gone out of the window a bit and people have felt confident to develop know- ledge...

He then wondered what doctors would eventually end up doing. The senior partner suggested that they would go to pieces or become adminis- trators.

In the Sanders Practice, where one of the practice nurses was very keen to develop her role along the lines of the nurse practitioner model, the partners suggested that it was very feasible that the practice would encou- rage this development, but they were in a state of flux, with one of the doctors retiring in the near future and the woman partner anxious to go full-time if she could. However, a strong note of caution on the limits of trust and confidence which doctors might place in the nurses was sounded by one of the doctors in this same practice. In the first group discussion he was anxious to stress how essential it was that there was a very good working relationship between doctors and the nurse practitioner, so that, as with the practice nurses, if they felt worried about something, they would not hesitate to bother or interrupt the doctor. By the time of the second group discussion, 15 months later, his position had shifted only a little:

> I was one who voiced this from the beginning as a valid concern ... I think we
> are very lucky in having [the nurse practitioner] ... she has always exercised
> strict self-discipline ... if she did not feel 100% about something, she came
> through and asked us or got extra help ... I would still think that there would
> be some nurses who are not best suited to nurse practitioner type work...

This point opened up a debate about the nature and adequacy of the
training available to nurses to allow them to practise as first-point-of-
contact nurse practitioners, and to enable them to transfer their skills.

It was clear from the discussions that the doctors in all the practices
were conscious that nurses (not just the nurse practitioner) could do much
of the work which they did. As one of the doctors in the Johns Practice
put it:

> ...I believe that many of the skills that I have are eminently acquirable by
> good practice nurses ... and I think that you could take any of the individuals
> in this room ... .and train them to do almost anything that I do, and do it
> equally well if not better ... but it takes time, and I think it has to be done a
> little bit at a time...

In the Sanders Practice they felt threatened by this and foresaw a shift in
government policy as this information came to light. This practice was
also the only one to be concerned about the medico-legal implications of
nurses' increased autonomy. They were careful to draw a distinction
between the trust they placed in *their* nurse practitioner and trusting a
nurse whom they did not know to practise safely.

In the Ongar and Johns Practices they reacted differently. In the former,
one of the doctors took some months to express his confidence in the
professional competence of the nurse and demonstrated this by checking
each patient carefully before agreeing to sign a prescription. But in this
practice the doctors came to see the nurse practitioner as a valuable additional resource in a hard-pressed practice, both for her general surgery
work and for her special knowledge of the problems of the menopause. In
the Johns Practice the doctors went further, by suggesting that the nurse
practitioner, and the other nurses, were no longer 'doing things' for the
doctors, but were allowed, and trusted, to get on with doing the things
that they were good at.

The picture here is a complex one, a different reaction from doctors in
each of the three practices, and within each practice, to the nurse practitioner. It cannot therefore be assumed, if other practices are anything like
the ones in the Derbyshire Project, that doctors would necessarily accept
or welcome the concept of a nurse running her own general surgeries or
agree on the implications of this for their practice.

What about the nurses themselves? The three nurse practitioners were
clear about the differences between their scope of practice as practice

nurses and as nurse practitioners providing a general surgery service. The move towards greater autonomy in professional practice had not been painless. They described their new work as much more taxing. All three had worried in the early days about missing an important symptom and making other mistakes. The nurse in the Ongar Practice described how, a year after starting her own surgeries, she still worried about missing something important, but that she found she was getting a 'gut reaction'* when she felt something was wrong.

The nurse practitioners were, however, unequivocally enthusiastic about their work and their new responsibilities. They enjoyed being able to 'go further' without referring to a doctor. They also derived satisfaction from having patients come back to them and from knowing that they had been able to help. This element of the nurse practitioners' job satisfaction, which derived from making someone feel better and an acknowledgement of that from patients, compares closely with the job satisfaction which the doctors said they got from playing a part and making a difference in the lives of their patients.

Although a significant proportion (in one practice it was about 50%) of nurse practitioner consultations resulted in drug treatment and the nurses were not able legally to sign prescriptions, they seemed to cope with the minimum fuss and inconvenience to patients by arranging for one of the doctors during surgery to sign a prescription on their behalf in between seeing patients. In contrast, the doctors in the Sanders Practice were having difficulty in encouraging their practice nurses, in the course of running their disease management clinics, to come through with prescriptions to sign. This was because the nurses did not feel comfortable with the notion that they were taking over responsibility from the doctors in deciding on particular drugs or strengths, even in the areas of chronic disease management in which they had trained and had recognized expertise.

These reactions suggest that this particular nursing role, providing a general surgery service and not knowing in advance what the patients are coming about, *is* different from the practice nurse role, including the situations, such as health promotion clinics, where the practice nurses are practising in an extended role. The reactions suggest that the issue of confidence, both of doctors in nurses and nurses in themselves, is an important one. There were examples in these three teams of nurse practitioners having less confidence in themselves than the doctors had in them and, conversely, instances of some of the doctors expressing wariness

---

*This phrase resembles Balint's 'flash of understanding' when a doctor, during a consultation, comes to a realization about a patient's condition, based on more than a hypothetico-deductive approach to the problem, by also encompassing the patient's perspective (Balint, 1957).

about extending the limits of their trust in nurses beyond the already recognized boundaries.

There was also a suspicion, expressed by the GPs in the Sanders Practice, of external training courses. Their concern was that a nurse trained as a nurse practitioner but unknown to them would not necessarily have their confidence and trust. This contrasts with the situation with practice nurses, and also within the medical profession, where GPs take on new partners on the basis of qualifications and do not suggest 'in-service' training. This suggests limits to the acceptability of this nurse practitioner model on the part of some doctors. It further suggests that the nurse practitioner role is indeed new, and with it therefore comes the whole raft of management of change issues of which trust and confidence are but two.

Role and employment status differences provide a further problem: nurses often move on while partners tend to stay. For nurse practitioner training and development this presents a difficulty. In the Sanders Practice the senior partner described the substantial investment in time which had been required to develop a nurse practitioner, and confessed that they would not have the capability 'in house' to start from the beginning again should the nurse practitioner leave.

It is a truism that all general practices are unique. It would therefore be fanciful to expect that the same perspectives would emerge from a study involving three practices. Equally, practices have much in common. A further examination of the themes elucidated above reveals that in the Derbyshire Project all three practices *shared* views on the following:

- pride in the quality and range of services which they provided

- concern expressed by the doctors about the pressures of managing the organization

- need for clarity in roles within the primary health care team

- acknowledgement of the overlap in roles between nursing and medicine in primary care

- ability of nurses within the primary health care teams to work together without duplicating roles

- the positive value of the additional appointments which the nurse practitioner service offered for patients

- the fact that the nurse practitioner consultations were less hurried

- the different kind of consultation which the nurse practitioner was able to offer through combining professionalism with a lay understanding developed through experiences which they had in common with patients

- the nurse practitioners' anxieties and enthusiasms about the new role

- the nurse practitioners' specializations in addition to the generic surgery consultation service.

The differences were as follows:

- *development of the nurse practitioner model*: the Ongar Practice provided a nurse practitioner consultation service which was close to the medical model, dealt with problems which would otherwise have been seen by the doctor and 'freed up' doctor time; the Johns Practice articulated a complementary model, with a focus on the development of roles according to what colleagues were best at and best suited to; the Sanders Practice also described a complementary model but talked of substituting for the doctor

- *role threat*: doctors in the Sanders Practice described how they felt threatened by the nurse practitioner role. This did not feature with the other two practices

- *trust*: doctors in the Johns Practice did not mention any concerns about the issue of trusting the nurse practitioner; one doctor in the Ongar Practice had concerns at the start; a doctor in the Sanders Practice had concerns about accepting a nurse in this role whom the practice had not trained in-house

- *job fulfilment for the nurse practitioners*: in the Ongar Practice the nurse practitioner expressed frustration at the lack of external training opportunities; in the Sanders Practice her main concern was the lack of recognition within the practice and outside for her new role; in the Johns Practice, the nurse expressed no barrier to job fulfilment.

As far as challenges within general practice are concerned, the double-edged sword for the doctors in all three practices was their pride in the quality of services provided combined with their concern about their capability to manage into the future. In considering changes in services to patients provided by the nurse practitioner role there was agreement across the three practices that the nurse practitioner provided valuable additional appointments to the surgery consultation service, that her consultation style was less hurried and that she offered a different kind of consultation. There was also a consensus in participants' views about the need for clarity about roles and an acknowledgement of overlapping roles between medicine and nursing and within nursing.

There was a difference in the way in which they described the development of the nurse practitioner model, with two focusing on a nursing model complementary to the doctors' function and a third developing a nursing model supplementing the doctors' function. Doctors in one practice saw the nurse practitioner as a potential threat. Participants who were doctors described different levels of difficulty in trusting a nurse working in this new way. Participants in two of the practices reported some degree of intraprofessional rivalry within nursing. Finally, the nurse practitioners themselves reported two different barriers to job fulfilment: unmet training needs, and formal and informal recognition.

Broadly speaking there was a convergence in views about the challenges within general practice and also about the impact of the nurse practitioner service on patient services, but a range of views about the impact of the nurse practitioner on the roles and relationships within the primary health care team and about the training issues.

One of the themes which emerged from the group discussions was the relative value placed on doctors' time and on nurses' time. The nurse practitioners described patients' concerns about taking up the doctor's time, to the extent, on occasion, of patients practising their own form of triage to check whether it was necessary to 'bother' the doctor. Two of the three nurse practitioners offered no additional comments of their own on this, but the third nurse indicated that she felt undervalued and that her time was precious too. There has been little work since Bowling on interprofessional relationships in primary care. Mackay, however, has studied relationships between doctors and nurses in the hospital setting and found that there are some highly influential variables affecting the way in which doctors and nurses see each other and work together (Mackay, 1993). She suggests that, among other factors, class, status, gender, training and education all affect the way in which nurses and doctors work together. The way in which the doctors and nurses contributed in the focus group discussions in the Derbyshire Nurse Practitioner Project and the comments on the value of the doctor's time would seem to bear this out. Mackay has described the hierarchical nature of nurse–doctor relationships in the hospital setting and the essential difference in the balance of power between the two professions, which she argues lies in the consultant's ultimate responsibility for patient treatment in hospital and the GP's responsibility for treatment outside hospital. However, despite this power imbalance, Mackay suggests that the cultural values of the two professions appear to be moving marginally closer as a result of the UKCC Code of Conduct, with its emphasis on personal responsibility and autonomous practice for nurses, and the development of audit and evaluation, which bears down on doctors' clinical freedoms (Mackay, 1993). The pressure to provide evidence-based care and treatment, and the need to work in teams rather than in isolation, could combine with an enhanced nursing role as nurse practitioner, and the greater confidence and assertiveness derived from this enhanced role, to change the power balance at the surgery. A further constraint in primary care is the financial and legal barrier to nurses being partners in general practice, but there is a signal from the centre that this has been recognized, with the new freedoms allowed by the NHS Primary Care Act 1997. Nurse partners could take ultimate responsibility for patient care alongside their medical colleagues.

There is one caveat to this equal sharing of responsibility for patient care: prescribing rights are still denied, so that every prescription that a nurse practitioner initiates must have a doctor's signature. In the Derbyshire Project and in others, this hindrance is mitigated thus: within the care and treatment protocols used by the nurse practitioners are prescribing policies encompassing the drug treatment of choice for a variety of problems. If a prescription is required the nurse practitioner prints it and takes it to a doctor, who signs it without seeing the patient. This can be organized fairly efficiently but still undermines the nurse's autonomy and wastes the time of patients and doctors. Under UK law nurses cannot prescribe except in nurse prescribing pilot sites. Many nurse practitioners, and indeed practice and district nurses, are involved in protocol schemes supplying prescription-only drugs. The implementation of nurse prescribing nationally, as well as expanding the existing formulary, would serve to legitimize the prescribing behaviour which many nurses are already involved in. It would also benefit patients, nurses and doctors.

There is one final question of status. Some nurses (for example, Johnson, 1997) would like to put an end to the employer–employee relationship and be full partners in the practice in which they work. If the nurse practitioner is indeed exercising professional autonomy, accepting and discharging patients into and out of the primary health care system, making decisions about diagnosis, treatment and management and is, in some organization models, responsible for the planning and delivery of care provided by all the primary care nursing team, this seems to be a reasonable development and request. Until recently, the Red Book regulations did not allow for this, but the 1996 White Paper *Choice and Opportunity* and the subsequent Primary Care Act 1997 removes this barrier. The White Paper notes that there are some positive disincentives for practices who want to replace a doctor with a nurse, even where this might be more efficient and provide better patient services. The legislation enables those who wish to do so to pilot different types of contract to test their practical implications and the benefits they could bring.

It has to be said that there has been no flood of applications for the employment status of nurses working in primary care to be changed since the passing of the 1997 Act. Just as some doctors are shying away from the lifelong commitment of a partnership, many nurses may not be ready to exchange the flexibility of the staff position for the responsibility of a partnership. There may also be socioeconomic reasons why a partnership position may not be a viable option for a nurse. But there are also undoubtedly cultural influences at work. How many nurses went into the profession with this end in mind? It will take some time and the emergence of more role models like Barbara Stilwell, who did go into a form of partnership with a medical colleague in the 1980s, for this career alternative to present itself as a realistic and achievable goal for nurses. Equally many doctors are ready to share power with nurses, but a large number are not. How many take comfort from the uniprofessional peer group 'feel' of the current partnership arrangements, where all members have been through the same initiation rites of medical school, exhausting junior hospital jobs and vocational training schemes? The professional and financial structures are now in place to allow a sea change in nurse–doctor relationships in primary care; the emergence of the nurse practitioner role will enable individuals to come forward to facilitate this change, but the process is likely to be slow.

Nurse practitioners and other nurses

How did the coming of the nurse practitioner affect the other nursing members of the team in the Derbyshire Project? If there was overlap in roles between the doctors and the nurses, there was undoubtedly also acknowledged overlap between the nurse practitioner and some of her colleagues within her own discipline, most notably the practice nurses and the health visitors.

In all the practices the nurses and doctors thought that there was some overlap in the kind of things which the nurse practitioner and the practice nurse did. It was pointed out at the second group discussion at the Sanders Practice that the practice nurses were developing their role in a similar way to the nurse practitioner: they too were getting to grips with the management of certain conditions and identifying the need to initiate and adjust drug treatments. One of the doctors in this practice provided an example of the limits to this role development on the part of the practice nurses (who were not present at the focus group discussions):

> ...They are enjoying it as well ... they can all manage asthma now as well as we can ... they haven't got to the stage of coming through with a prescription yet ... and I say to X; 'Why don't you bring a prescription for me to sign?' And she said, 'I think it is presumptuous of me' ... I said, 'No, it isn't ... you know what we are going to do ... why don't you bring it and I'll sign it ... I haven't disagreed with anything you have done yet...'

In the Johns Practice they had come to the conclusion that the nurse practitioner/practice nurse distinction was artificial; if they were completely different, one of the doctors said, they would not be able to ask their nurse practitioner to carry out some of the traditional practice nursing jobs which she was doing part of the week. In the Ongar Practice the nurse practitioner had developed an interest in menopause and HRT, but it was likely that one of the practice nurses would have fulfilled that role if it had not been for the advent of the nurse practitioner; and one of the doctors explained that there was a growing trend for many chronic conditions to be monitored out of normal surgery and he often referred patients to the specific clinics run by the practice nurses as well as the menopause clinic run by the nurse practitioner.

Nearly all the other nurses pointed out other similarities between what they did and some of the things that the nurse practitioner did, particularly the way in which patients used practice nurses, district nurses and health visitors to get more information and advice about health problems. Duplication of roles was anticipated by the health visitors in the Ongar Practice in the first group discussion. In particular, there was a concern that the nurse practitioner was carrying out the same function in the surgery as they were in the home with young children. The health visitors also expressed the hope that they would get more referrals from the nurse practitioner as time went on. By the second group discussion there had not been much growth in referrrals from the nurse practitioner to the health visitors, although there had been a steady stream the other way. But one of the health visitors saw the dynamics of the team in a slightly different way from nine months earlier:

> There are a lot of skills which we underuse because we haven't the time to do everything we would like to do. There are potential overlaps in all the roles but I don't see that as a problem because we can all work together and do whatever we are able to do ... whatever we most want to do ... out of the skills that we have got ... there is no shortage of work...

A similar situation was reported in the Sanders Practice, where there had been long-term understaffing on the health visiting side and where the health visitors, rather than accepting referrals from the nurse practitioner, had become accustomed to asking her to do the follow-up on their behalf.

In the Johns Practice two-way referrals between the health visitors and the nurse practitioner were more evenly balanced. They reported more discrete areas of expertise, with the health visitors receiving referrals to see children and the nurse practitioner receiving referrals on women's health issues. The relationship with the district nurse was also closer: they helped each other out on days off, while acknowledging each other's area of expertise when both were in. In the other two practices little contact was reported between the district nurses and the nurse practitioners.

In all three practices the comment was made that in many aspects, although there was potential overlap, there was in fact little overlap in responsibilities within the nursing teams. In chronic disease management, for which both practice nurses and nurse practitioners had responsibilities, they had specialized in different areas. For example, in the Ongar Practice the practice nurse ran the asthma clinic, whereas in the Sanders Practice it was the nurse practitioner. In the Ongar Practice the nurses talked about their roles running alongside each other. In the Sanders Practice, however, the doctors reported that the nurses were keen to develop and train in the way in which the nurse practitioner had done: one wanted to go on the nurse practitioner diploma course at Manchester University and both wanted the opportunity to sit in on doctor–patient consultations. The tutorial system that had been developed to train the nurse practitioner within the practice was already beginning to be used to train practice nurses in greater depth in their areas of chronic disease management.

The practice nurses in the Ongar and Sanders Practices were mildly envious of the attention and status accorded to the nurse practitioner. In the Ongar Practice, for example, one of the practice nurses made it clear that she would have become the practice 'expert' in menopause problems if the nurse practitioner had not come along. In the Johns Practice the practice nurse was emphatic that she operated in an extended role in a similar way to the nurse practitioner; for example, patients asked her for advice when they did not want to talk to the doctor. This nurse was also concerned that the particular model in place was tending too much towards the 'medical model', apeing what doctors did and not practising nursing. She was concerned as well not only about the rise of a 'mini-doctor', but of a nurse-technician type in primary care, and that tradi-tional nursing roles would get 'pushed out of the way'. Interestingly, this diminution or dilution of the 'nursing' component of the job was also the fear of the nurse practitioner in the Sanders Practice, expressed particularly in the first round of group discussions. She was quite clear that she did not want the role to develop as a sort of 'second-class doctor'. Was this 'sour grapes'? This seems unlikely, as the nurse practitioner in the Johns Practice also touched on this issue when she talked about not being very busy and worrying that patients would see her as the equivalent of the plumber's mate, and that they would want to see the plumber.

The health visitors were more perturbed about the nurse practitioners encroaching on their territory, and with the added advantage of having a prescription pad to hand. In fact, in two of the practices, because they were hard-pressed and short-staffed, the health visitors had begun to take advantage of the availability of the nurse practitioner. They had found that their clients welcomed the opportunity to see a nurse at the surgery without having to worry about whether their child's problem was 'serious' enough for the doctor. The nurse practitioner had also acquired useful skills, for example, in checking chests to see whether an infection had cleared. In the third practice the nurse practitioner and the health visitor had more discrete areas of expertise, the former focusing on women's health and the latter on children, so that it had not been difficult to work out a *modus operandi*.

The disruption caused by the nurse practitioner joining the other nursing members of the team was not perhaps as great as might have been expected. In two of the three practices it was the role, and not the person, that was new. Certainly there was minimal duplication, because the workload seemed to be distributed among them sensibly, even though there were potential overlaps in roles and definite overlaps in skills. There was also a feeling that the other nurses were watching to see if the scheme worked, and there was a sense that they wanted it to succeed because they shared some of the assumptions that lay behind it, in particular that nursing skills were being underutilized. What also emerged, however, was that they wanted their own contribution to primary care acknowledged and valued, and they had no intention of being 'left behind' by some new 'supernurse'.

The nurses in the Derbyshire study demonstrated that they were conscious of hierarchy and status. They also demonstrated sensitivities about the extended nursing role leading to a 'second-class doctor' or 'technician' model. But there was an acceptance, because patients were benefiting, of the nurse practitioner acting as a first-point-of-contact health professional and therefore also an acceptance of the new tasks of history taking, examination, diagnosis and management that the new role necessarily brought with it. The study suggests that nurses are preoccupied with issues of status and of professionalization and that this will affect the acceptability to them of the nurse practitioner role. Where improvements in services to patients can be successfully argued, nurses are likely to favour the new role.

It is also worth considering not only professional relations between nurse practitioners and other nurses working in primary health care, but also organizational ones. There has been an unhelpful split in the primary health care team for a long time between employed nursing staff (practice nurses and nurse practitioners, where they exist) and attached nursing staff (employed by the local community trust). Nurses themselves have worked hard to overcome this divide, but inevitably tensions have arisen over the years around the boundaries of areas of responsibility. One example is the annual health checks for the over-75s, which is a district nursing responsibility in some practices and a practice nurse responsibility in others. Fundholding and the purchaser–provider split have helped by clarifying, through the contracting process, the expectations of all parties. In some regions, the local trust has assumed responsibility for providing practices with all nurse services, including the practice nurse role, thereby relieving hard-pressed GPs of their recruitment and management responsibilities in the area of practice nursing. In other regions, the integrated nursing team approach has gained ground. The aim in this model is a relatively self-contained practice with a nursing team leader to coordinate the whole team, that is, the practice nurses, district nurses and health visitors. Operating within the constraints of statutory requirements, the nurses, after appropriate training, cover for each other, while retaining and developing their specialist skills. This approach can capitalize on existing strengths within the nursing team, particularly the close working relationships and flexibility about roles. It is easier to implement when there is not a high turnover of staff. The nurse practitioner, who is often the most highly trained of the nurses, sometimes assumes the role of nurse coordinator to this integrated team.

In the Derbyshire Nurse Practitioner Project, in the Johns Practice, the nurse practitioner has gone on to provide this nurse coordination role, and in the Ongar Practice the nurse practitioner manages the practice nurses. Care has to be taken that this person has not only the clinical expertise but also the management expertise and adeptness at interpersonal relations to undertake this role. It should be emphasized that it does not have to be the nurse practitioner who provides the nurse coordination for the team; and unless this nurse has the requisite skills, the other team members may resent this 'supernurse' and prefer management by a doctor (one of the GPs) or arms-length management by the trust.

6 Practical steps

Professional bodies as facilitators

This book has argued that the nurse practitioner, a new kind of nurse who can offer an alternative consultation service for patients, including diagnosis and treatment of minor illness, has a valuable part to play in British primary care of the future. Individuals taking on this role, and education courses to prepare them, are springing up all over the country. However, there is still no central steer from government or professional bodies, so that it is left to the enthusiasts and innovators among practitioners and educators to carry this forward. What more could be done to facilitate a comprehensive dissemination of good practice in the employment, training, deployment and development of nurse practitioners? First, perhaps alone among the professional bodies, the approach of the RCN has been forward thinking. In the 1980s the RCN provided indemnity cover for Barbara Burke-Masters and Barbara Stilwell and continues to provide cover for nurse practitioners working in their extended roles. In the 1990s the RCN started the first nurse practitioner diploma course, which for the first time provided successful students with a recognized and portable qualification, as well as the first cadre of nurse practitioner graduands and a larger group than before available for research and evaluation purposes. Annual nurse practitioner conferences run by the RCN also provide an opportunity for research briefings and networking, problem sharing and problem solving. The only drawback in all this is that the nurse practitioner concept could be seen as merely of 'nursing' interest. Indeed, non-nurses writing about nurse practitioners have been few, and policy makers at local and national level are also largely silent on the issue. The RCN now needs to imbue others outside nursing with the same enthusiasm about the nurse practitioner concept.

There is another body within nursing which is more equivocal about the concept; the UKCC has yet to recognize the title of nurse practitioner. As we have already seen, this means that anyone undertaking the job falls outside the UKCC's framework of registered, specialist and advanced practitioners, and therefore outside the safeguards and development opportunities provided by that framework. This is clearly an untenable situation:

on the one hand we have a highly respected nursing institution – the RCN – running education courses for nurse practitioners, and on the other we have the national regulatory body established by Parliament refusing to recognize the title. One or other must give way in the interest of safe patient care and the credibility of the profession. Of course, the role is more important than the title, and few would disagree that the words 'nurse practitioner' are misleading within the NHS and fairly meaningless to the layperson. Perhaps it is possible to recognize the role but come to a consensus about the title, although it must be said that both the role and the title have survived for over 30 years in the US.

The third professional body with a potentially valuable part to play is the RCGP. A number of prominent individual GPs have spoken out in favour of the concept and initiated experimental nurse practitioner projects; figures as diverse as Tudor Hart, of 'Inverse care law' and *A New Kind of Doctor* fame (Hart, 1971, 1988), Martin Roland, from the National Primary Care Research and Development Centre in Manchester, and David Colin-Thome, the Total Purchaser GP from Runcorn, are all involved. It would now be useful to hear a position statement from the RCGP on issues such as the training of nurse practitioners and their prospects as partners in the general practice of the future.

Another group that should take an interest is that representing managers in the NHS. Health authorities, which appear from the 1997 White Paper to have secured a permanent position in the 'new NHS', are likely to remain manager led. These powerful organizations, while supporting the development of primary care groups, will still allocate resources to them and hold them to account, as well as having responsibilities for deciding on the range and location of health care services. The Institute of Health Services Managers (IHSM) has for many years run a successful series of 'Medicine for Managers' courses; perhaps now is the time to consider 'Nursing for Managers'. The NHS Confederation, representing health authorities and trusts, may also wish to turn its attention to the availability and skills of nursing as well as medical manpower in primary care.

The groups mentioned here are powerful change agents; those interested in developing the nurse practitioner should seek to inspire the enthusiasts within these bodies so that they can act as facilitators in implementing some of the painful cultural changes necessary for nurse practitioners to become a mainstream component of primary health care provision.

Should every patient have access to a nurse practitioner?

We have seen from the Derbyshire Project, as from other studies in the UK and elsewhere, that generalist primary care nurse practitioners are popular with patients and provide high levels of patient satisfaction. The Derby-shire study found in particular that half the patients who had gone to see the nurse once went back to her within 12 months, despite high levels of accessibility to a doctor's appointment. This study also showed higher levels of satisfaction with the nurse consultation in comparison with the medical consultation with the respondent's usual doctor. Overall care given by the nurses was rated higher than the overall care given by the doctors. More women respondents consulted the nurse practitioner than did men or children, and also compared the experience more favourably.

On the face of it, a general conclusion is that in all three practices the respondents liked this nurse practitioner model of care. From a patient's viewpoint of the quality of care, therefore, it would appear that the research suggests a wider implementation of this model in primary health care.

But what was it about the nurse consultation that they appreciated? Because the patient surveys contained only structured questions, there was no oppportunity to ask *why* the respondents liked seeing the nurse, beyond the high satisfaction scores for explaining, listening, information, time and overall care. Would a practitioner from another profession who was good at these things do as well or better? Should we retrain doctors to concentrate more on these areas? Further clues came in the small number of statements in the 'any other comments' section where respondents remarked on the nurse practitioner's pleasantness, capacity for understanding and the fact that she was a woman. On the other hand, one person did not like being offered an appointment to see a nurse when she had telephoned to make arrangements to see the doctor. The findings from the primary health care team focus groups provide some further substantiation of the sentiments expressed in the 'any other comments' section. The nurses and doctors themselves thought that patients appreciated the more relaxed style of consultation the nurse was able to offer, the fact that she was a woman and, because of her background, had a greater degree of shared life experi-ences. But one nurse provided an echo of the respondent's criticism about being offered an appointment with the nurse when a doctor appointment had been requested, by likening herself to a 'plumber's mate'. None of this adds up to a detailed answer to what it is about the nurse–patient interaction in first-point-of-contact care that makes it acceptable and effective from the patient's perspective, and where the limits to that acceptability may lie. Patients from a later study on the Johns Practice identified nurses' dedication, technical skill and capacity for coordination as three key strengths of the members of the primary health care nursing team (Chambers, 1995). It is likely that it was these same strengths that the respondents appreciated about the nurse practi-tioner in the three participating practices.

Patients have always wanted quick access to the doctor. It has been suggested that a nurse practitioner may be the answer to some of the time pressures facing doctors, and from an organizational viewpoint the findings to date indicate that a nurse practitioner surgery consultation service, as additional provision rather than replacement for doctor appointment slots, *may* shorten the waiting time to get a doctor's appointment (Horder, 1996).

The absence of an unequivocal finding on this point is corroborated by other research touching on the same issue. An RCGP study from the late 1960s (reported in Bowling, 1981) showed that doctor–patient consultation rates decreased in surgeries that began to employ practice nurses, and that doctors used the extra time available to carry out other practice-related duties. But the evaluation of the South Thames Regional Health Authority nurse practitioner pilot projects (Touche Ross, 1994:42) did not find any tendency for the introduction of nurse practitioners to reduce the rate of consultation of patients, and in three of the six sites surveyed, there was a tendency for the overall rate of consultation of all kinds to rise, because of additional consultations with the nurse practitioner.

Despite the growth of teamworking in primary care and significant increases in numbers of practice nurses (six times as many in 1993 as in 1983; Department of Health, 1994), the General Household Survey indicates a very slow but steady increase in consultation rates with the GP, from an average of four consultations per year in 1972 to five in 1992, and a corresponding rise from 12% to 15% in the proportions who had consulted a GP in the 14 days before interview (OPCS, 1994).

It would not therefore be sensible at this stage to proceed with wholesale implementation of a nurse practitioner service solely on the basis that patients' access to doctors' appointments will improve. It seems likely that nurse practitioners, particularly in practices with large lists, high consultation rates or partners with substantial outside commitments, will initially help to fulfil some unmet demand, both by seeing patients themselves and by freeing up appointment time for doctors. This would undoubtedly entail a net additional cost On the other hand, if demand for health care is not in fact infinite and nurse practitioner hours in a practice were to increase over time, there would eventually be a falling off in demand for doctors' appointments.

The argument about the nurse practitioner fulfilling unmet demand may also explain why the Derbyshire Project found that the presence of the nurse practitioner service did not improve the quality of the medical consultation from the respondents' point of view. If the doctor was as pressurized as before because more patients were going through the system, he would be unlikely to change consulting behaviour, that is, to listen better, explain things more, and provide information and time, the four aspects of the consultation that were scrutinized in the research.

There may be another explanation. What we do not know is what doctors' potential is for improving their performance in these areas. The hypothesis was posed that with the new service doctors would have more time and would be seeing fewer patients with minor illness and more patients with clinically more complex problems more appropriate to their level of training and skills. The hypothesis has not been supported by the Derbyshire study. It may be that the medical style of working, developed over some years and in the context of general practice, is not amenable to change in the simplistic way envisaged. Inglis suggests that a more radical reappraisal of the mechanist medical model is overdue and that it is unlikely that the profession will change its ways fast enough to serve the community's requirements (Inglis, 1981).

On a more optimistic note, but also more wide-ranging than the one-change intervention of the nurse practitioner, Tudor Hart advocates the development of six features of medical professionalism as an alternative to the Osler paradigm. These include admitting what is not yet known and cannot be done, the imaginative rather than uncritical application of scientific principles, an understanding of disease and health as existing on one continuum rather than as separate entities, recognizing the skills of other health professionals in the effective conservation of health, treating patients as colleagues, and a more dependable alliance with the people served by doctors (Tudor Hart, 1988). Nurses may have much to offer in working with doctors to develop these features of medical professionalism, not least in rephrasing it as *clinical* professionalism, but it would be misguided to consider the introduction of a nurse practitioner service on its own as a means of improving the quality of the GP consultation.

To summarize the arguments from the patients' perspective: the research showed, first, that the respondents liked the nurse practitioner service; second, that access to doctors' appointments was largely unchanged; and third, the presence of the nurse practitioner was not associated with improvements in the quality of the GP consultation. Should government policy with regard to the potential contribution of nurse practitioners in primary care change in the light of this? The answer to this will be clearer after a consideration of the professional perspective.

The research found that the primary health care teams involved in the project welcomed the model with some reservations. The doctors recognized that the nurses were able to push back the boundaries of their scope of practice. They respected their levels of skill and consistency of approach, and they felt confident that the nurses would be able to recognize the limits of their expertise. They thought that the patients appreciated the enhanced choice of care at the first point of contact because the model offered the opportunity for care by a woman and a nurse.

There were three major points of concern, all expressed by doctors in the Sanders Practice, the only one which was not a training practice. First, if the model was introduced throughout the NHS, they argued that it would put doctors out of work. Second, the doctors said that they trusted 'their' nurse because they already knew her, but they were not sure whether they would have allowed the same scope to a nurse who was unknown to them, even if she had been on an appropriate training course. Third, although their confidence in the nurse was partially based on the fact that she had carried out much of her training for this role at the practice, they also complained that the training had been a heavy burden on them. Abel-Smith describes a situation which echoes this one, at the beginning of the 20th century, when nurses were struggling to gain registration and some of the doctors were worried that this process would result in work being taken away from them (Abel-Smith, 1960).

The three nurse practitioners were all excited by their new role and the improved services which they felt they were able to give to patients. Each had a different reservation. In the Ongar Practice the nurse was concerned that there was a limit to her professional development without an opportunity for a college-based theoretical qualification supporting the role. In the Johns Practice there was a sense that patients still preferred to see a doctor, although this sense had diminished by the time of the second focus group. In the Sanders Practice the nurse felt undervalued for the work she did.

The other community nurses also welcomed the model, although there had been some initial suspicion and resentment. These nurses had had feedback that the patients liked being able to see the nurse practitioner as an alternative. They also considered that although there could be an overlap in roles, there was more than enough work for everybody, and that what was required and what they felt they had done, was to allocate responsibilities, for example, for particular client groups such as young children, in a logical fashion according to resources and need. Their main concern was that they did not want to be considered 'second division', and to be left behind by some 'supernurse'. Their argument here was that they also operated to some degree as nurse practitioners, not in terms of first-point-of-contact care, but in their area of expertise.

From the perspective of the health professionals in the three Derbyshire practices the model was found to be acceptable. For some doctors there were issues surrounding the possible threat to their role, the problem of not being able to trust nurses and the training burden. For the nurse practitioners the issues included the lack of opportunities for formal courses, the lack of self-worth and the sense of being undervalued. For the other nurses in the primary health care teams the main issue was one of a threat of perceived professional inferiority. What are the lessons for the future development of primary care? Should every patient have access to a nurse practitioner?

On the negative side, studies thus far have not demonstrated that introducing nurse practitioners would be a panacea for all the current major problems in general practice. Some of these need to be tackled urgently, but not by the introduction of a nurse practitioner. There is no evidence from this study that having nurses working alongside doctors in first-point-of-contact care improves the quality of the doctor consultation. It is also possible that in many practices, the introduction of the nurse practitioner may uncover unmet demand for consultations and therefore it could be costly. The study suggests that some doctors would be resistant to the model because of the threat to their professional position and their lack of confidence in the nursing profession to take on some aspects of first-point-of-contact care.

On the positive side, respondents rated the quality of the nurse practitioner consultation service and the overall care which she gave highly. There was also some evidence that the new service may have improved accessibility to see the doctor. The primary health care teams involved welcomed the model, including the doctors who had entrusted some of their first-point-of-contact care responsibilities to the nurses, the nurse practitioners who had taken on the new role and their colleagues who fitted into and worked with the new model. The conclusions must be that this model has benefits. However, it does not address all the key problems of primary care, particularly the quality of the doctor consultation and the increasing pressures faced by GPs. It would also need careful handling when it comes to more extended implementation.

The studies do provide some clues for prioritizing wider implementation. Women particularly welcome the opportunity to consult with a practitioner of their own gender. There is evidence that more women GPs are being trained: over half of the GP trainees in 1993 were women. However, the trend towards equal proportions of full-time male and female GP principals is slow: by the same year only 26% of principals were women and only three quarters of them were full-time (Department of Health, 1994). It would therefore seem logical to consider, as a high priority, the introduction of nurse practitioners in practices with no female partner. As the research shows for this to be a viable complementary consultation service, it would also make sense to introduce these nurses in practices where this might be most required, for example, in areas of greatest deprivation, with high consultation rates and poor access or take-up of health promotion. Nurse practitioners, including those in this study, have tended to be nurtured by innovative practices who have volunteered to take risks. If Tudor Hart's inverse care law pertains, these practices are likely to be serving the least deprived populations (Tudor Hart, 1971). These nurses should be introduced into practices with single-handed practitioners or where the teams are under the greatest stress. The one setting out of the three in this study where there was equal availability of a nurse practitioner and a doctor (the Sanders Practice, where the nurse practitioner operated from the branch surgery) was the one where the doctors felt the most benefit in terms of difference to their workload. It was also the practice where the nurse practitioner scored most highly in patient satisfaction in the patient surveys. Horder recommends that, in any event, the division of labour between doctor and nurse practitioner is best decided in the place of work, rather than in the councils of professional representative organizations (Horder in Meads, 1996).

The Derbyshire study also sheds light on issues in the marketing of the nurse practitioner role. There were three areas of difference between the professionals' predictions and their experiences of the nurse practitioners' impact on patients. First, the take-up of the service by parents for the care of minor illness presented by their children was notable. Second, professionals reported that patients welcomed the opportunity to consult with an experienced and highly skilled health professional who also shared common lay experiences with them and spoke their 'language'. Third, there was a problem with the terminology; patients sometimes tended to confuse 'nurse practitioner' with either the GP or the practice nurse. These issues would need to be dealt with to ensure that patients for whom the service was intended had a clear understanding of what the nurse practitioner was able to offer.

Would it work? There is a widespread precedent, in relation to the pregnant woman, which could usefully be adapted for generalist first-point-of-contact care by nurses. The midwife is often now the lead carer for pregnant women and also the first point of contact when something goes wrong (Chambers, 1995b). There is growing evidence (for example, Mellor and Chambers, 1995) that this model of care is highly acceptable to women, as long as there is access to the doctor if necessary. It is generally acceptable to doctors, although there is some regret about the loss of contact and continuity of care.

To summarize, if health authorities want to invest where nurse practitioners would 'add maximum value' to the quality of the primary health care service, there are a number of features of existing provision to look out for. *High list sizes* indicate doctors under stress and difficulty for patients in obtaining access to an appointment. A nurse practitioner service would obviously alleviate the problem. If there are areas where it is *difficult to fill partner vacancies*, a replacement by a nurse practitioner could be considered. *High consulting rates*, often in areas of deprivation, also cause stress for doctors and access problems for patients. *Practices without a female partner* and *single-handed practices* both limit choice for patients; a nurse practitioner service would again be beneficial. Finally, the

Derbyshire study and a later project in Runcorn have demonstrated the particular benefits of a nurse practitioner located in a *branch surgery*.

How practices can make the nurse practitioner model work

A nurse practitioner surgery consultation service clearly can bring benefits to practices. In particular, it can allow hard-pressed GPs to get on with other work and provide an enhanced choice for patients, and can challenge nurses who would like to work in an extended role. For all that, it seems unlikely that any lead or push is going to come from the centre to carry this idea forward, since ministers and civil servants have in the 1990s been more preoccupied with the internal market and, as the century turns, are now set to be focused on commissioning by primary care groups and on health improvement programmes. In the absence of guidance 'from above', how can practices who are interested make a success of this initiative? The following tips are drawn from a combination of sources: personal experience in establishing a nurse practitioner service in three practices; contact with, and desk research about, other nurse practitioners, and time spent as a health service manager followed by a decade in management consultancy in primary care. The advice should be treated with appropriate caution.

The first point is to *gain the support of the health authority*. This is important for a number of reasons: the health authority can be helpful when it comes to meeting training needs, sorting out local professional concerns and for financial reasons, because health authorities are often keen to be associated with innovative projects which can demonstrate better services for patients and successful professional development. It is likely that the introduction of a nurse practitioner service will cost more money: they will be an additional service, and these nurses can be expensive (they are usually paid on G or preferably H grade), and initially their training needs – particularly if they attend a nurse practitioner diploma course – will be expensive. Financially, the trade-off is that, in the longer term, savings can be made. Again health authorities may be interested in exploring this; some practices with nurse practitioners are able to operate with higher-than-average list sizes or to take on more outside paid work (for example, medico-legal work, occupational health sessions, hospital clinical assistantships, commissioning work) than would otherwise be the case. In these scenarios the nurse practitioner has become a doctor substitute, and it may well be that the practice would like to invite the nurse to be a partner. As the Red Book regulations do not allow for this, the practice would need to apply to be a Primary Care Act Pilot (PCAP), and the health authority would be able to act as a guide on this.

A new nurse practitioner service needs *the commitment of all the part-ners*. We have seen that doctors' attitudes to nurses taking on some of their tasks vary greatly, from unbounded enthusiasm to outright hostility. It would be unwise to embark on a nurse practitioner service if one or more of the partners were hostile: it puts the nurse in an impossible posi-tion and sets the partners themselves on a collision course. Some honest exploratory discussions within the partnership are therefore recommended, perhaps on a partners' 'away day' when options for the future direction of the practice are being considered. It is unlikely that all the partners will be as keen as the one (if the suggestion comes from a doctor) who first proposes the idea. In each of the three Derbyshire practices discussed in detail in this book there were 'doubters' as well as 'enthusiasts'. But all the partners were willing to give it a go; they were convinced that patients and themselves might indeed benefit by the additional service.

Beyond the commitment of partners to this particular initiative, it is worth asking whether, within the practice as a whole, there is a *culture of innovation*. This may include a record of risk taking and challenging the norm without necessarily being 'leading edge'. Stocking argues that there are a number of preconditions for successful change in the wider NHS, of which general practice could be seen as a microcosm (Stocking, 1988). First, is the climate of opinion right? This includes not just the partners but, for example, the other nurses who would be working alongside, receiving referrals from and referring to the nurse practitioner; the trust who may employ the district nurses and health visitors; and the health authority who may be needed for support and investment. Second, are there enthusiastic local champions? The history of nurse practitioners in the UK suggests that at least one nurse and one doctor in each practice should be articulate ambassadors to persuade others within the organiza-tion and sceptics outside it. Third, the change (in this case the new nurse practitioner service) should meet a need. All change is difficult, messy, painful and time consuming, and the evidence from the studies described in this book is that introducing nurse practitioners is no exception. It is important therefore that there is a problem or need in the practice which a nurse practitioner service might address. As we have seen earlier, the problem might be a high list size per doctor, high consulting rates, needy patients from a deprived area (for which the health authority may be persuaded in the interests of equity to fund additional support), a branch surgery with little doctor cover or the absence or shortage of female prac-titioners. Stocking also argues that it makes sense for the change to be an 'add-on' rather than something totally new. For example, it would not work where the practice nurse role was a relatively new concept. The change is unlikely to be successful if it is seen as incompatible with roles, attitudes and routines, if it is complex to organize and thought to bring relatively little benefit. If significant local stakeholders are convinced that these factors hold true, the practice will have difficulty pursuing the change. Stocking found that changes are easier to implement if there is little explicit additional finance required, but that lack of money is rarely the key obstacle, because if people are keen enough they solve the funding question (Stocking, 1988).

Having decided that the preconditions are favourable, it is important to *plan the implementation*. This includes spelling out the anticipated benefits to patients and staff, identifying how the new service will be evaluated (does it yield the anticipated benefits?) and how it is planned that the change will affect the work of the doctors. It is important that if the new service is geared to 'free up time' for doctors as well as meet a 'care gap', the doctors are clear what they will do with the time so that they can 'feel' as well as demonstrate the benefit. In order not to set it up to fail, there needs to be a reasonable timescale for each of the main steps: disseminating the proposal internally and externally, recruitment, training, shadowing, protocol development, date for 'going live', review markers, and initiation and completion of interim and final evaluation schemes.

One of the early tasks is to *sort out the medico-legal aspects* of a nurse working in an extended role. There are two parts to this: the first is addressing concern on the part of partners about 'letting go' and about placing trust in a non-medical colleague, and the second involves checking out the continuing validity of the professional indemnity insurance with the nurse's and the doctors' defence or representative bodies. These organizations will normally require a copy of the job description as a minimal requirement. All practices have an obligation to make sure that any employee is suitably trained for the job in hand. Nurses themselves are legally liable if they fail to exercise the skills normally expected of them or if they undertake tasks that they are not competent to perform. As the employer, the doctor may also be vicariously liable. The nurse has the ultimate responsibility for deciding whether she is competent for a particular task and must refuse delegation if she feels it is inappropriate; this invidious situation can always be avoided if there are mutually agreed training programmes and decisions about competence. In general, the nurse should only take on new tasks when she feels ready, when there has been appropriate training, preferably documented, and the doctor also agrees that the nurse is competent in that area.

Drawing up and *agreeing the job description* is a critical stage in the successful management of this change. It is helpful if 'ownership' of the job description is as widespread as possible, not only by the partners; comments should also be invited from the other nurses, perhaps also the trust and the health authority. A model job description is provided in Figure 6.1.

The *recruitment process* should include drawing up a person specification as well as the job description so that the practice knows before inter-

Figure 6.1   Nurse practitioner model job description.

Title: nurse practitioner
Responsible to: partners of the practice
Hours of work:

Job summary
To provide an alternative surgery consultation service for patients, working closely with the general medical practitioners, and focusing particularly on minor illness, general health advice and information. The post is initially for a fixed period only. Training will be provided, and continuing assessment by one of the partners, in the role of mentor. The post-holder will be expected to assist in the evaluation of the project.

Main responsibilities
1. To see patients by appointment or without an appointment who present for diagnosis, treatment or advice

2. To carry out examinations, make diagnoses and arrange treatments within the post-holder's competence, within protocols as agreed with the partners, and under the guidance of the mentor

3. To provide telephone advice to and triage for patients requiring a 'same day' appointment

4. To triage on-call requests for home visits at times agreed with the partners but not between midnight and 0800

5. To provide information, advice and reassurance to patients

6. To acquire and use knowledge and skills about the diagnosis and treatment of minor illnesses for the benefit of the patients of the practice

7. To acquire and use counselling knowledge and skills for the benefit of the patients of the practice

8. To provide patients, practice staff and other members of the primary health care team with up-to-date information on the role of the nurse practitioner to maximize appropriate use of her skills

9. To keep the necessary records for practice management purposes and for the purposes of evaluating the project

10. To assist with the development and evaluation of the project, for example, by sharing and resolving problems with the other nurse practitioners

views start what kind of nurse is being sought. It is likely that only a nurse with some significant primary/community experience would be appropriate. Partners may also wish to stipulate a minimum educational qualification, so that they know that the nurse is able to cope with the academic challenges of a diploma course, if it is intended that the nurse should attend such a course. It may be useful to have a nurse manager from the trust, nurse adviser from the health authority or nurse practitioner from another practice as an external assessor. It is useful to go through the interview stage even when the practice is proposing to appoint from among existing staff, for example, the practice nurse, district nurse or health visitor. This gives the nurse and the partners the opportunity to discuss and agree the new role, to offer and to accept (or reject) the new position.

Following the appointment, a *training needs assessment* should be drawn up with the successful candidate. Health authority staff could provide advice here. A plan for how and when the training needs will be met should then be devised. One area for debate is agreeing how much training can take place 'on the job', that is, after the nurse practitioner has started to act as an alternative consultant and to provide her own surgeries, and what essential skills are required before this moment. It is not necessary to have completed a one-year training programme before starting surgeries, but the extent to which the nurse is able to operate autonomously is limited by the extent of her knowledge in dealing with problems presented by patients. In the early days, therefore, much more of her workload may have to be checked by, referred to or shared with a doctor than will be the case later on. This may sound time consuming, but in fact patients appear to choose appropriately between nurse and doctor (as long as there is a choice) and therefore duplication of effort is minimized.

One of the problems for the newly appointed nurse practitioner can be professional isolation, and having a *doctor mentor* chosen from one of the partners can be immensely useful. This person may organize tutorials, help with protocol development, and act as a source of comfort and support at what can be a challenging time, perhaps the most challenging of a nurse's career. The mentor can also negotiate the 'shadowing phase' with their colleagues. Nurses in the Derbyshire Project found it useful to 'shadow' doctors (that is, to sit in on doctor consultations) and then have the doctors shadow them before running their own surgeries. Some doctors, particularly those not in training practices, find this phase unnerving because they have grown unused to someone observing their clinical practice. In a group partnership it is valuable for the nurses to sit in on all the partners' surgeries to gain experience of varied consulting styles and to witness how different kinds of patients choose to see different kinds of doctors. The mentor should continue as a source of support after the nurse has begun her own surgeries and as time goes on, provide advice on audit and evaluation of the new role. The nurse will also need a nursing colleague to provide intraprofessional clinical supervision; this may be someone from a trust, health authority or working in nurse education.

Throughout the training period and when plans are being drawn up for 'going live', it is vital to establish *ongoing dialogue with the other nurses in the practice and also other staff*, particularly receptionists. Sharing some of the processes of *protocol development* can be a valuable catalyst in teambuilding, resolving potential conflicts and avoiding misunderstandings. It is best not to be too overambitious with protocols or to rely on them to cover all combinations or variations on health problems in primary care, but to start with the two to three most common presenting minor illness problems in the practice and work from there. It is likely that other nursing colleagues will have valuable comments or additions to make to the protocols. Receptionists must be convinced that offering the alternative of an appointment with a nurse practitioner can be a choice genuinely valued by patients and not a 'second-class' option because there are no doctor appointments left. Receptionists therefore need to understand what the nurse has to offer and why patients may find it useful to see them.

Receptionists can also help with *marketing the concept with patients*; an explanatory leaflet and advance notice of the new service are important. Just as when a new partner starts, that doctor tends at first to be less busy until they have built up a list of 'their patients', so it may take time for the new service to be fully taken up. Where there is an acute shortage of doctor appointments or no access to a female practitioner apart from the traditional practice nurse sessions, this is less likely to happen and the nurse practitioner may find herself very busy very quickly. Other colleagues also have a part to play in explaining the new service: district nurses and health visitors can suggest an appointment with the nurse practitioner for their client or member of their family if they think it appropriate.

Starting up a new service is a unique opportunity to conduct a 'before and after' study as part of an *evaluation*. Because the nurse practitioner caseload and speed of working is likely to change over time, it is a good idea to start collecting data from the outset. Support in researching the effects of the nurse practitioner role may be available locally from a university, medical school or college of nursing or through the health authority. The evaluation should focus on examining the extent of those effects of the new intervention which were the main reasons for introducing it in the first place. General patient acceptability of, and patient satisfaction with, the nurse practitioner service are now well documented; less well covered in research in the UK are the relevance of training programmes to practice, differential clinical outcomes of nurse practitioner and general practitioner consultations, the impact of the length of consultation time on patient satisfaction with nurse practitioners, and quantitative differences in doctor workload before and after the inception of the nurse practitioner role. Other interesting research challenges include disproving the hypothesis that nurse practitioners 'feed' an infinite demand for surgery consultations, and assessing the impact of nurse practitioners on the nature of the workload of GPs. Further work on the nature of the nurse–patient relationship would be useful. Finally, exploring the changes in intranursing relations and doctor–nurse relations would be helpful in identifying an optimal nurse–doctor skill-mix for the future for primary care.

References

Abel-Smith B (1960) *A History of the Nursing Profession*. Heinemann, London.

Age Concern (1986) *GPs and the Needs of Older People: A Policy Paper*. Age Concern, London.

Annandale-Steiner D (1979) Unhappiness is the nurse who expected more. *Nursing Mirror* 29 November: 34–6.

Baker R (1990) Development of a questionnaire to assess patients' satisfaction with consultations in general practice. *British Journal of General Practice* 40:487–90.

Balint E, Courtenay M, Elder A, Hull S and Julian P (1993) *The Doctor, the Patient and the Group*. Routledge, London.

Balint M (1957) *The Doctor, His Patient and the Illness*. Pitman, London.

Bliss A and Cohen E (eds) (1977) *The New Professionals*. Aspen Systems Corporation, Maryland.

Bowling A (1981) *Delegation in General Practice: A Study of Doctors and Nurses*. Tavistock, London.

Bowling A and Stilwell B (eds) (1988) *The Nurse in Family Practice*. Scutari Press, London.

Brown S and Grimes D (1995) Meta-analysis of nurse practitioners and nurse midwives in primary care. *Nursing Research* 44(6):332–9.

Buchan I and Richardson I (1973) Time study of consultations in general practice. *Scottish Health Studies No 27*. Scottish Home and Health Department.

Buchan J (1996) Nurse shortages (editorial). *BMJ* 312:134–5.

Butterworth CA (1991) Setting our professional house in order. In: *Nurse Practitioners: Working for Change in Primary Health Care Nursing* (ed J Salvage), King's Fund, London.

Calman M and Williams S (1991) Please treat me nicely. *Health Service Journal* 17 January: 25.

Cartwright A (1983) *Health Surveys in Practice and in Potential: A Critical Review of Their Scope and Methods.* King's Fund, London.

Cartwright A and Anderson R (1981) *General Practice Revisited.* Tavistock, London.

Chambers L, Burke M, Ross J and Cantwell R (1978) Quantitative assessment of the quality of medical care provided in five family practices before and after attachment of a family practice nurse. *Canadian Medical Association Journal* 118:1060–4.

Chambers N (1995a) Report on a study to obtain a patients' and carers' perspective of the nursing services provided by the Darley Dale primary health care team. Unpublished.

Chambers N (1995b) Users' views of antenatal maternity services in the community: a report for Northamptonshire Family Health Services Authority. Unpublished.

Chambers N (1996a) Practice visions. *Primary Care Management* 6(2):11–12.

Chambers N (1996b) Nurse practitioners in primary care: an alternative to a consultation with the doctor ? University of Manchester, PhD thesis.

Chambers R and Belcher J (1993) Work patterns of general practitioners. *British Journal of General Practice* 43:410–12.

Cohen P (1984) Nurse practitioner in East London. *Nursing Times* 80(2):22–4.

Colwill J (1992) Where have all the primary care applicants gone? *New England Journal of Medicine* 326(6):387–92.

Department of Health (1989) *General Practice in the NHS.* HMSO, London.

Department of Health (1989) *Report of the Advisory Group on Nurse Prescribing.* HMSO, London.

Department of Health (1992) *Health of the Nation.* HMSO, London.

Department of Health (1994) *Statistical Bulletin: Statistics for General Medical Practitioners in England and Wales 1983–93.* HMSO, London.

Department of Health and Social Security (1971) *Organisation of Group Practice.* HMSO, London.

Department of Health and Social Security (1986) *Neighbourhood Nursing – A Focus for Care* (Cumberlege Report). HMSO, London.

Department of Health and Social Security (1986) *Primary Health Care: An Agenda for Discussion*. HMSO, London.

Department of Health and Social Security (1987) *Health Services Development: Community Nursing Services and Primary Health Care Teams*. HMSO, London.

Devereaux M (1991) NPs in North America. In: *Nurse Practitioners: Working for Change in Primary Health Care Nursing* (ed J Salvage), King's Fund, London.

Diers D and Molde S (1983) Nurses in primary care: the new gatekeepers. *American Journal of Nursing* 83:742–5.

Dubos R (1968) *Man, Medicine and Environment*. Pall Mall Press, London.

Fawcett-Henesy A (1992) The development of the NP in primary care. *Primary Health Care Management* 2(13):9–11.

Fry J (1992) *General Practice: The Facts*. Radcliffe Medical Press, Oxford.

Fry J and Horder J (1994) *Primary Health Care in an International Context*. Nuffield Provincial Hospitals Trust, London.

General Medical Council (1993) *Tomorrow's Doctors: Recommendations on Undergraduate Medical Education*. GMC, London.

General Medical Services Committee (1991) *Your Choices for the Future*. British Medical Association, London.

Gordon P and Hadley J (eds) (1996) *Extending Primary Care*. Radcliffe Medical Press, Oxford.

Grogan S, Conner M, Willits D and Norman P (1995) Development of a questionnaire to measure patient satisfaction with general practitioner services. *British Journal of General Practice* 45:525–9.

Hammer M and Champy J (1993) *Re-engineering the Corporation*. HarperCollins, New York.

Holmes G *et al.* (1976) Contribution of a nurse clinician to office practice productivity. *Health Services Research* II(I):1–33.

Honigsbaum F (1979) *The Division in British Medicine*. Kogan Page, London.

Horder J (1996) The international context. In: *Future Options for General Practice* (ed G Meads), Radcliffe Medical Press, Oxford.

Howie J, Porter A, Heaney D *et al.* (1991) Long to short consultation ratio: a proxy measure of quality of care for general practice. *British Journal of General Practice* **41**:48–54.

Hughes J (1996) The managed practice. In: *Future Options for General Practice* (ed G Meads), Radcliffe Medical Press, Oxford.

Huntington J (1995) *Managing the Practice: Whose Business?* Radcliffe Medical Press, Oxford.

Hutchinson E (1963) *General Practice: A Consumer Commentary.* Research Institute for Consumer Affairs, London.

Illich I (1976) *Limits to Medicine.* Marion Boyars, London.

Inglis B (1981) *The Diseases of Civilisation.* Hodder and Stoughton, Sevenoaks.

Irvine D (1993) General practice in the 1990s. *British Journal of General Practice* **43**:121–5.

Jacoby A (1989) *User Surveys of General Practice.* Institute for Social Studies in Medical Care, London.

Johnson W (1997) The nurse practitioner in primary care. *Primary Care* **7**(4):10–12.

Jones P (1984) The Canadian experience. *Nursing Times* 335–41.

Kassirer JP (1994) What role for nurse practitioners in primary care? *New England Journal of Medicine* **330**(3):204–5.

Kaufman G (1996) Nurse practitioners in general practice: an expanding role. *Nursing Standard* **11**(8):44–7.

Kirwan M and Armstrong D (1995) Investigation of burnout in a sample of British general practitioners. *British Journal of General Practice* **45**:259–60.

Lancaster J and Lancaster W (1993) Nurse practitioners: health care providers whose time has come. *Family and Community Health* **16**:2.

Law S and Britten N (1995) Factors that influence the patient centredness of a consultation. *British Journal of General Practice* **45**:520–4.

Lewis JR and Williamson V (1995) Examining patient perceptions of quality care in general practice. *British Journal of General Practice* **45**:249–53.

Mackay L (1993) *Conflicts in Care: Medicine and Nursing.* Chapman and Hall, London.

McBride M and Metcalfe D (1995) GPs' low morale: reasons and solutions (editorial). *British Journal of General Practice* 45:228–9.

McKeown T (1979) *The Role of Medicine*. Blackwell, Oxford.

Martin P (1991) Nurse practitioners. *Pulse* 16 November: 85–93.

Mauksch IG (1978) The nurse practitioner movement – where does it go from here? *American Journal of Public Health* 68(11):1074–5.

Mead G (ed) (1996) *Future Options for General Practice*. Radcliffe Medical Press, Oxford.

Mellor J and Chambers N (1995) Addressing the patient's agenda in the re-organisation of antenatal and infant health care: experience in one general practice. *British Journal of General Practice* 45:423–5.

Miles A (1991) *Women, Health and Medicine*. Open University Press, Milton Keynes.

Miller DS and Backett EM (1980) A new member of the team? *Lancet* 358–61.

Mundinger M (1994) Advanced practice nursing: good medicine for physicians? *New England Journal of Medicine* 330:3.

Munro K and Gibbs T (1997) Time out. *Health Service Journal* 1 May:30–1.

National Association of Health Authorities and Trusts (1994) *Partners in Learning*. NAHAT, Birmingham.

NHS Executive (1994) *Developing NHS Purchasing and GP Fundholding: Towards a Primary Care-led NHS*. HMSO, London.

NHS Executive (1996) *Primary Care: The Future*. HMSO, London.

NHS Executive (1997) *The New NHS White Paper*. The Stationery Office, London.

Neal R *et al.* (1996) Frequent attenders: who needs treatment? *British Journal of General Practice* 46:131–2.

Office of Health Technology Assessment (1986) *Nurse Practitioners: A Policy Analysis*. Health Technology Case Study 37, Washington.

O'Meara D (1994) Alberta nurse practitioner loses suit with college about right to practise. *Canadian Medical Association Journal* 150(8):1294.

OPCS (1992) *General Household Survey*. HMSO, London.

Patients' Association (1973) *Patients and their GPs*. Patients' Association, London.

Pendleton D (1995) Professional development in general practice. *British Journal of General Practice* 45:377–81.

Petchey N (1994) Exploratory studies of GPs' orientations to general practice and responses to change. *British Journal of General Practice* 44:551–5.

Petersdorf R (1992) Primary care applicants – they get no respect. *New England Journal of Medicine* 326(6):408–9.

Poulton B (1995) Keeping the customer satisfied. *Primary Health Care* 5(4):16–19.

Pratt J (1995) *Practitioners and Practices: A Conflict of Values?* Radcliffe Medical Press, Oxford.

Pritchard P and Pritchard J (1994) *Teamwork and Shared Care*, 2nd edn. Oxford University Press, Oxford.

Read S and Graves K (1994) *Reduction of Junior Doctor Hours in Trent Region: The Nursing Contribution.* University of Sheffield, Sheffield.

Rice G (1990) *Understanding Doctors*. Michael Joseph, London.

Riley J (1998) *Helping Doctors Who Manage*. King's Fund, London.

Ritchie J, Jacoby A and Bone M (1981) *Access to Primary Health Care*. HMSO, London.

Robinson G, Beaton S and White P (1993) Attitudes towards practice nurses: survey of a sample of general practitioners in England and Wales. *British Journal of General Practice* 43:25–9.

Robinson R *et al.* (1997) Cracks in the edifice. *Health Service Journal* 4 September:26–8.

Rosenthal M (1995) *The Incompetent Doctor*. Open University Press, Buckingham.

Rout U and Rout JK (1993) *Stress and General Practitioners*. Kluwer Academic Publishers, Lancaster.

Royal College of General Practitioners (1994) *Education and Training for General Practitioners*. RCGP, London.

Royal College of General Practitioners (1996) *The Nature of General Medical Practice*. RCGP, London.

Seabrook M, Booton P and Evans T (1994) *Widening the Horizons of Medical Education*. King's Fund, London.

Sharron H (1984) Nurse practitioner with a mission. *Primary Health Care* 2(9):14–15.

Shurin S (1993) Letter. *New England Journal of Medicine* 329(1):728.

Sox H (1979) Quality of patient care by nurse practitioners and physician's assistants: a ten year perspective. *Annals of Internal Medicine* 91:459–68.

Spitzer W *et al*. (1974) The Burlington randomised control trial of the nurse practitioner. *New England Journal of Medicine* 290:251–6.

Spitzer W (1984) The nurse practitioner revisited: slow death of a good idea. *New England Journal of Medicine* 310(16):1049–51.

Stilwell B (1982) The nurse practitioner at work. *Nursing Times* 78:1799–803.

Stilwell B (1984) The nurse in practice. *Nursing Mirror* 158:17–19.

Stilwell B (1988) Nurse practitioners in British general practice. In: *The Nurse in Family Practice* (eds A Bowling and B Stilwell), Scutari, London.

Stilwell B (1991) An ideal consultation. In: *Nurse Practitioners: Working for Change in Primary Health Care Nursing* (ed J Salvage), King's Fund, London.

Stilwell B *et al*. (1987) A NP in general practice. *Journal of the RCGP* 37(297):154–7.

Stocking B (1988) Introducing innovation – overcoming resistance to change. In: *The Nurse in Family Practice* (eds A Bowling and B Stilwell), Scutari, London.

Stott N (1994) The new general practitioner (editorial). *British Journal of General Practice* 44:2–3.

Touche Ross (1994) *Evaluation of Nurse Practitioners Pilot Projects*. Touche Ross, London.

Tudor Hart J (1971) The inverse care law. *Lancet* i:405–12.

Tudor Hart J (1988) *A New Kind of Doctor*. Merlin Press, London.

United Kingdom Central Council for Nursing, Midwifery and Health Visiting (1992) *The Scope of Professional Practice*. UKCC, London.

United Kingdom Central Council for Nursing, Midwifery and Health Visiting (1994) *The Council's Proposed Standards for Post-registration Education.* UKCC, London.

Vuori H (1987) *Patient satisfaction – attribute or indicator?* Proceedings of an International Symposium on Quality Assurance in Health Care. Joint Commission on Accreditation of Hospitals. WHO, Geneva.

Warden J (1988) Rise of the nurse practitioner. *BMJ* **296**:1478.

Watkins C (1981) *The Measurement of the Quality of General Practitioner Care.* RCGP, London.

Which? (1987) Making your doctor better. May: 230–3.

Which? (1995) What makes a good GP? June:18.

Williamson V (1988) *GP Services: Mothers' Views.* Brighton Community Health Council, Brighton.

World Health Organization (1978) *Alma Ata Declaration.* WHO, Geneva.

Wysocki S (1990) Rural health care: a challenge and opportunity for nurse practitioners. *Nurse Practitioner Forum* **2**(2):68–70.

Further reading

Ambrose D (1986) GPs still oppose prescribing by practice nurses. *Pulse* **46**(37): 16.

Ashburner L *et al.* (1997) *Nurse Practitioners in Primary Care: The Extent of Practice and Research.* Centre for Health Planning and Management, Keele University.

Atkin C and Hirst M (1994) *Costing Practice Nurses: Implications for Primary Health Care.* University of York, York.

Barber JH and Kratz CR (1980) *Towards Team Care.* Churchill Livingstone, Edinburgh.

Blaxter M and Paterson E (1982) *Mothers and Daughters. A Three Generational Study of Health Attitudes and Behaviour.* Heinemann, London.

Bosanquet N (1991) Lessons for future policy. In *Nurse Practitioners: Working for Change in Primary Health Care Nursing* (ed J Salvage), King's Fund, London.

Brown P (1995) Minor injuries – major advance. *Nursing Management* 2(2):8–9.

Bryden P (1992) The future of primary care. In: *Continuity and Crisis in the NHS* (eds R Loveridge and K Starkey), Open University Press, Buckingham.

Campbell S (1997) Nurse practitioners at the cutting edge of today's NHS. *Primary Care* 7(8):2–4.

Carey L (1995) Practice nurse or nurse practitioner? *Primary Health Care* 5(9):2–14.

Chambers N (1987) Developing a consumer strategy in the NHS or getting things right. *Hospital and Health Services Review* January: 12–14.

Chambers N (1993) Final report on the GP practice-based survey report for Northamptonshire Family Health Service Authority. Unpublished.

Chew R (1995) *Compendium of Health Statistics*, 9th edn. Office of Health Economics, London.

Cochrane AL (1972) *Effectiveness and Efficiency*. Nuffield Provincial Hospitals Trust, London.

Cornwell J (1984) *Hard-earned Lives*. Tavistock, London.

Damant M, Martin C and Openshaw S (1994) *Practice Nursing*. Mosby, London.

Department of Health (1995) *The Patients Charter and You*. HMSO, London.

Dowrick C, May C, Richardson M and Bundred P (1996) The biopsychosocial model of general practice. *British Journal of General Practice* 46:105–7.

Expert Group on Maternity Care (1993) *Changing Childbirth*. HMSO, London.

Fairkurst K, Stanley I and Griffiths C (1995) Should medical students learn more about management? *British Journal of General Practitioners* 45:2–3.

Feig P (1988) A content analysis of health-related information in a popular woman's magazine – Woman's Own. University of Manchester, MSc thesis.

Fenton M, Rounds L and Anderson E (1991) Combining the role of the nurse practitioner and the community health nurse. *Journal of the American Academy of Nurse Practitioners* 3(3):99–105.

Giles S (1993) Partner potential. *Nursing Times* 89(38):62–63.

Handy C (1985) *Understanding Organisations*, 3rd edn. Penguin, Middlesex.

Handy C (1989) *The Age of Unreason*. Random Century, London.

Head S (1988) The new pioneers. *Nursing Times* **84**(26):27–8.

Hill J (1986) Patient evaluation of a rheumatology nursing clinic. *Nursing Times* **82**(27):42–3.

Hunt G and Wainwright P (eds) (1994) *Expanding the Role of the Nurse. The Scope of Professional Practice.* Blackwell Scientific Press, Oxford.

Jefferys L, Clark A and Koperski M (1995) Practice nurses: workload and consultation patterns. *British Journal of General Practice* **45**:415–18.

Jefferys M and Sachs H (1983) *Rethinking General Practice.* Tavistock, London.

Jordan S (1993) Nurse practitioners, learning from the USA experience: a review of the literature. *Health and Social Care* **2**:173–85.

Khayat K and Salter B (1994) Patient satisfaction surveys as a market research tool for general practices. *British Journal of General Practice* **44**:215–19.

Lenehan C (1994) Nurse practitioners in primary care – here to stay? *British Journal of General Practice* **44**:291–2.

Mackay L (1989) *Nursing a Problem.* Open University Press, Milton Keynes.

Mahoney DF (1992) A comparative analysis of nurse practitioners with and without prescriptive authority. *Journal of the American Academy of Nurse Practitioners* **4**(2):71–6.

Marsh G (1993) Achieving the full potential of the primary health care team. *Primary Health Care Management* **3**(1):5–7.

Marsh GN and Dawes ML (1995) Establishing a minor illness nurse in a busy general practice. *BMJ* **310**:778–80.

McDowell HM (1984) Family nurse practitioner. *International Nursing Review* **31**(6):177–9.

Mellor H (1992) The Derbyshire NP scheme – the first nine months. Unpublished.

NHS Executive (1995) *An Accountability Framework for GP Fundholding.* HMSO, London.

Nettleton S (1995) *The Sociology of Health and Illness.* Polity Press, Cambridge.

Ngcongco N (1991) Lessons learnt in Botswana. In: *Nurse Practitioners: Working for Change in Primary Health Care Nursing* (ed J Salvage), King's Fund, London.

O'Connor CA (1993) *The Handbook of Organizational Change.* McGraw-Hill Europe, Maidenhead, Berks.

Openshaw S (1984) Literature review: measurement of adequate care. *International Journal of Nursing Studies* 21(4):295–304.

Ovretveit J (1992) *Health Service Quality.* Blackwell Scientific Publications, Oxford.

Polgar S and Thomas S (1991) *Introduction to Research in the Health Sciences.* Churchill Livingstone, Melbourne.

Price M *et al.* (1992) Developing national guidelines for nurse practitioner education. *Journal of Nursing Education* 31(1):10–15.

Read S (1994) Do formal controls always achieve control? The case of triage in Accident and Emergency Departments. *Health Services Management Research* 7(1):31–42.

Richman J (1987) *Medicine and Health.* Longman, Harlow.

Robinson J, Gray A, Elkan R (eds) (1992) *Policy Issues in Nursing.* Open University Press, Milton Keynes.

Royal College of Nursing (1985) *Written Evidence to the Committee of Enquiry into Nursing* (Cumberlege Report). RCN, London.

Salisbury C (1991) Working in partnership with nurses. *British Journal of General Practice* 41:398–9.

Salisbury C and Tettersell M (1988) Comparison of the work of a nurse practitioner with that of a general practitioner. *Journal of the RCGP* 38:312, 314–26.

Salvage J (ed) (1991) *Nurse Practitioners: Working for Change in Primary Health Care Nursing.* King's Fund, London.

Salvage J (1992) The new nursing. In: *Policy Issues in Nursing* (eds J Robinson, A Gray and R Elkan), Open University Press, Milton Keynes.

Scott M and Marinker M (1993) Imposed change in general practice. *BMJ* 30(7):1189.

Tattam A (1987) A practical service. *Nursing Standard* 2(11):32.

Tomson P (1991) Editorial. *British Journal of General Practice* 41:45–7.

Trnobranski P (1994) Nurse practitioner: redefining the role of the community nurse? *Journal of Advanced Nursing* 19:134–9.

United Kingdom Central Council for Nursing, Midwifery and Health Visiting (1991) *Report on Proposals for the Future of Community Education and Practice.* UKCC, London.

Walby S, Greenwell J, Mackay L and Soothill K (1994) *Medicine and Nursing: Professions in a Changing Health Service.* Sage, London.

Watson P, Hendey N and Dingwall R (1994) *Role Extension/Expansion with Particular Reference to the Nurse Practitioner.* University of Nottingham, Nottingham.

Webb R and Hannay D (1996) Career choices of trainees in general practice. *BMJ* 312:314.

Whitcomb M and Desgroseilliers J (1992) Primary care medicine in Canada. *New England Journal of Medicine* 326(22):1469–72.

Wilkin D (1986) Outcomes research in general practice. *Journal of the RCGP.* 36:4–5.

World Health Organization Study Group (1994) *Nursing Beyond the Year 2000.* WHO, Geneva.

Wright S (1995) Sales pitch for nursing's softer side. *Nursing Management* 2(2):16–18.

Appendix A

Derbyshire NP Project: list of questions used in patients' questionnaire and correspondence with hypotheses under test

Q1   How many times have you consulted the doctor in the past 12 months?

Q2   How soon can you get an appointment? *(Null hypothesis #1: The presence of a nurse practitioner makes no difference to patient waiting times for an appointment compared with the absence of a nurse practitioner)*

Q3   Is that reasonable?

Q4   How long do you have to wait at the surgery? *(Null hypothesis #2: The presence of a nurse practitioner makes no difference to patient waiting times in the surgery compared with the absence of a nurse practitioner)*

Q5   Is that reasonable?

Q6   How well would you say that you know the doctor?

Q7   How well does he listen? *(Null hypothesis #3: The presence of a nurse practitioner makes no difference to patient satisfaction with doctor consultations compared with the absence of a nurse practitioner)*

Q8   How good is he at explaining things? *(Null hypothesis #3: see above)*

Q9   How much information does he give you? *(Null hypothesis #3: see above)*

Q10 Do you have enough time with him? *(Null hypothesis #3: see above)*

Q11 How would you describe the care you get from your doctor? *(Null hypothesis #4: The presence of a nurse practitioner makes no difference to patient satisfaction with overall care given by the doctor compared with the absence of a nurse practitioner)*

Q12   How is your health?

Q13   Are you a man or a woman?

Q14   How old are you?

Q15   Who owns your home?

Q16   Any other comments

E1   How often have you consulted the nurse practitioner?

E2   How well does she listen? *(Null hypothesis #5: There is no difference between patient satisfaction with consultations with the doctor and consultations with the nurse practitioner)*

E3   How good is she at explaining things? *(Null hypothesis #5: see above)*

E4   How much information does she give you? *(Null hypothesis #5: see above)*

E5   Do you have enough time with her? *(Null hypothesis #5: see above)*

E6   How would you describe the care you get from the nurse practitioner? *(Null hypothesis #6: There is no difference between overall patient satisfaction with care given by the doctor and care given by the nurse practitioner)*

Appendix B

Derbyshire NP Project: summary of hypothesis tests and results

Variables (participating practices only)	Round 1	Round 2	Total	Chi-square	P value
Waits for appt less than 24 hours (Hyp #1)	250	255	505	0.048	>0.8
Waits less than 10 minutes (Hyp #2)	89	87	176	0.02	>0.8
Dissatisfaction counts with medical consultation (Hyp #3)	170	139	309	3.22	>0.05
Care = Excellent from doctor (Hyp #4)	96	110	206	0.62	>0.3

Round 1 = Absence of nurse practitioner

Round 2 = Presence of nurse practitioner

Variables	GPs	NPs	Total	Chi-square	P value
Dissatisfaction counts with consultation (Hyp #5)	58	22	80	16.2	<0.001*
Care = Excellent (Hyp #6)	51	72	123	4.3	<0.05*

Null hypothesis #1: The presence of a nurse practitioner makes no difference to patient waiting times for an appointment compared with the absence of a nurse practitioner

Null hypothesis #2: The presence of a nurse practitioner makes no difference to patient waiting times at the surgery compared with the absence of a nurse practitioner

Null hypothesis #3: The presence of a nurse practitioner makes no difference to patient satisfaction with doctor consultations compared with the absence of a nurse practitioner

Null hypothesis #4: The presence of a nurse practitioner makes no difference to patient satisfaction with overall care given by the doctor compared with the absence of a nurse practitioner

Null hypothesis #5: There is no difference in patient dissatisfaction between nurse practitioner consultations and general practitioner consultations *Null hypothesis overturned*

Null hypothesis #6: There is no difference in patient satisfaction with overall care given by the nurse practitioner and overall care given by the general practitioner *Null hypothesis overturned*

Appendix C

Derbyshire NP Project: comparisons between respondents. The women's, children's and men's experiences of the consultation and overall care

Consultation dissatisfaction counts	GPs	NPs	Total	Chi-square	P value
Women n = 110	40	13	53	11.79	<0.001*
Children n = 28	7	3	10	0.4	>0.5
Men n = 51	11	6	17	0.52	>0.3
Total n = 189	58	22	80	16.2	<0.001*
Care = Excellent counts	GPs	NPs	Total	Chi-square	P value
Women n = 110	27	39	66	1.5	>0.2
Children n = 28	8	14	22	0.72	>0.3
Men n = 51	16	19	35	0.28	>0.8
Total n = 189	51	72	123	4.3	<0.05*

Index